THE
PHOENIX
CHILD

Also by Henry Viscardi, Jr.

A MAN'S STATURE '52
GIVE US THE TOOLS '59
THE SCHOOL '64
A LAUGHTER IN THE LONELY NIGHT '61
A LETTER TO JIMMY '62
THE ABILITIES STORY '67
BUT NOT ON OUR BLOCK '72
The Phoenix Chd '74

Henry Viscardi, Jr.

THE
PHOENIX
CHILD

A Story of Love

Paul S. Eriksson, Inc.
New York

For Edwin J. Beinecke, Jr.
whose friendship is exceeded only
by his love for our
wonderful children

Contents

Preface

This is a story of love.

The cast of characters is as unlikely as you could find in America, and yet it is all a part of this wonderful country. It is the story of a legless man, a pretty Jewish girl and her family, and a small black boy.

There are hundreds of other characters in this story, and none of them are bit players. There are the scores of devoted people who have helped make a dream come true. There are other scores of handicapped who have been involved in one way and another. There are doctors and nurses, and social workers, and a compassionate judge. It is a story of patience and devotion and quiet heroism. It is a story of medical marvels that have been and are being performed to save a soul. Above all it is the story of hope and a look into the future.

Henry Viscardi, Jr.

Albertson, New York
August, 1975

THE
PHOENIX
CHILD

I

Darren

I was in the gymnasium watching the kids play basketball.

Suddenly an object skittered across the floor and came to a halt right next to the little electric cart I was riding. I looked down. It was a human eye. Brown.

Just then a small black boy came charging up breathlessly, picked up the eye, and started to clap it back into the socket on the left side of his face.

"Hey!" I shouted.

"That's all right, Dr. Viscardi," he grinned. "Happens all the time. It's still a little loose."

"No" I said. "That's not what I meant. Did you ever hear of hygiene?"

"Sure! Miss Singleton is always talking about it."

"Well, one thing it means is we don't spit on our eye and stuff it back in after it's been on the gym floor. Come on, let's go up to the nurse's office."

So I started up my cart and the two of us moved out of the gym and along the corridor of the school building to the office of Judy Davidson, our school nurse. She took the eye from me, washed it in the little sink, without a word, and handed it to the boy. He calmly put it into place, looked at me for approval and, when I nodded, he went scampering off back to the basketball floor.

Well, Judy," I said, "he certainly doesn't seem to let things upset him very much, does he?"

She laughed. "Not Darren. You know, Dr. Viscardi, it's hard to realize that he is the same little boy who came in here three years ago."

I thought about that for a moment. She was right, and she did not even know how right, for just that day Headmaster Dick Switzer of the school, Miss Singleton, who is Darren's first grade teacher, and I had been talking, and if Judy would agree, we were going to approach the Syosset school authorities to see if they would take Darren Dillard into second grade next fall. Here was a boy who had come to us as a grotesquely disfigured young child, a discard of society, and within four years he was going back into the mainstream of American life. He would go to school, and —unless I missed my guess by a mile—he would make it just fine. He would grow up and probably go on to college and do with his life just what he wanted to do without frustration or fear for the future. The Darren Dillard story is what our school at Human Resources is all about, and it is the kind of tale that fills every one of us with hope and with the satisfaction that we are doing the job we made for ourselves.

Looking at this well-built, healthy seven-year-old, I could hardly match him up in my mind with the scrawny little scared rabbit that had come to us three and a half years before. And frightened half to death. There was reason enough for it—he had been pushed around, from one institution to another, in one foster home and then another, until it was a wonder that he was able to respond to anything.

Little Darren Dillard. What a change!

Martha, his mother, was a young black woman who lived with her mother in one of those big public-housing apartment complexes in the Bronx, the ones you see standing stark and ugly, as you head along the Cross Bronx Expressway on your way to the Throg's Neck Bridge. It was poor and ugly, and a blight on the face of New York, but it was the way it was. Martha was on welfare, and she had been since the birth of her first child, Linda, eight years earlier when she was sixteen years old. Linda was a pretty little child and she grew fast. Three years later Martha had another child. He was a healthy baby, too, and active. Martha's husband soon deserted her and she moved in with her mother then, into a bigger apartment in the same building. The growing family needed space and Martha's mother needed the help with the rent and grocery money.

Then one night Martha went to a dance out on

Long Island where she met a man. She had an affair with him and two months later she found out she was pregnant. In February, 1968, Martha went to the hospital with labor pains.

Early on the morning of February 9, they took her into the delivery room and later there was a slapping noise, and a loud wail from a tiny baby boy.

Martha did not see the doctor's face. He must have frowned and shaken his head, and when the nurse took the little brown baby from him, she winced, then cuddled him into his little blanket, rocked him for a moment and laid him down in the bassinet to be wheeled to the sterile, glassed room that was the hospital nursery.

The doctor had frowned and the nurse had winced because what they saw was a disfigured little head. The baby had no left eye, nor a left ear at all. The hairline grew right down the left side of his face as though no ear had been intended. He had a cleft palate and a hare lip.

"Poor little fellow," said the nurse in charge of the nursery station. "What kind of a life can he have in store for him?" She shook her head dolefully.

No one prepared Martha for the shock. When she woke up from the anesthetic, a nurse stuck her head in the door, saw that she was stirring, and said "I'll get your baby."

That was standard procedure. The nurse who said it did not know—she was a floor nurse, not from the pediatrics department. She went to the nursery. The nurse in charge shook her head slowly once again and picked up the baby to carry him to his mother, dreading the task ahead. Shielding the baby's left side, she brought him into his mother, and laid him down on the pillow. Martha picked him up, looked, gave a little cry and began to sob. The nurse comforted her. In a few minutes it was all right. The baby began to suckle noisily.

But it was not all right two days later when Martha's mother came to visit her daughter. Martha's mother was an inveterate reader of the New York *Enquirer* and a follower of astrology. When she saw the baby she became dreadfully upset, and put her head down on the bed and began to cry. Her sobbing became so pronounced that an intern was called and gave her a sedative. When she had quieted, she told Martha and the nurse that she had felt the most dreadful worries ever since Martha read in the paper that a Gemini of Martha's birthdate would have bad luck during February, and that a child born on February 9th was going to be unlucky. And there it was—look how it had turned out! She pleaded with Martha to leave the baby at the hospital.

What a dreadful plight that must have been for poor Martha. For even though she now knew the problems she must face, she loved the baby. But she loved her mother, and she saw clearly that to keep the little baby she was going to have to go through a veritable maze of troubles. I was not there of course, but I have seen so many women like Martha. She was a good woman, and, having four children of my own —all daughters—I know how she must have felt. Because of her personal situation, and her fears and feelings of inadequacy in dealing with this little baby, she was simply not equipped to care for him with his many special problems.

The first of these became apparent in the very early days in the hospital. Little Darren could not nurse properly because of his cleft palate and hare lip. They took him away and began giving him special feedings. Martha knew, after a few days, that she was going to leave little Darren with the hospital. Not breastfeeding him made it easier.

Martha was in the hospital for a week. Not until she left did she tell her doctor that she could not take the baby. He was sympathetic, but the administrators not so much so. They cajoled and pressed, but Martha's mother was as strong as they and she knew what a hard life it would be for all of them, especially little Darren. Martha was badly torn, but in the end she weighed her own difficulties and decided that she must stick with her decision. So she left the hospital and went back to the apartment without the baby.

When Darren was two weeks old the doctors operated on his harelip for the first time and gave him an almost normal mouth. It would take another operation, but that could not be done for a year or so, until the tissues had set. At least he could drink properly. Still he had no left eye, nor any sign of an ear.

Deformed. Unwanted. Black.

Such a baby did not seem to have much chance in life.

2

Shuttled

If you are to understand the miracle of Darren Dillard you must have some picture of the life he lived before he came to the Human Resources School on Long Island. For in the beginning society seemed to conspire in negative behavior against this helpless little boy in a way that threatened to turn him into a useless person. There are useless persons—they are made by inhuman treatment unleavened with love. And in his first three years of life, little Darren's existence was very short on love indeed.

After the baby had been six months in the hospital, he had outgrown the facilities and the administrators were complaining that the hospital could not bear the expense further. He must be turned over to the city authorities and treated as a waif, put into an institution, or in some way handled so that he would stop being an expense to the nursery. Really, little Darren was in no shape to go anywhere; his cleft palate and his harelip were only partly repaired. He was not the most handsome of babies, without ear or eye. He needed treatment and love.

He got neither.

He was sent to the foster home of Mrs. Carrie Brown in the Bronx. Mrs. Brown was a favorite of the welfare department; she was a big black woman in her fifties, a woman who had raised children of her own. She lived in a six-room attached house on Weaver Street. I know a dozen women like Mrs. Brown—they are honest women doing a job that society demands, taking care of foundling children from birth through infancy. But when you are caring for four or five, changing diapers, making formula, washing, bathing and cleaning up, and keeping house and making ends meet and doing the shopping and trying to take care of yourself, you do not have much time left over. Nor at the end of a day is there much time and energy for love in your life. Mrs. Brown was a decent woman. She did not beat the children or mistreat them in any way. Sometimes she might lose her temper, as would any mother, foster or real. But the real mother would make up for it with love, with little hugs and kisses, a tickling session in the playpen. A child at home would be surrounded with rattles and dolls, and his playpen would be pulled out into the sunny part of the living room in the morning.

Not Darren's.

He had no playpen. His crib was lined up against the wall of the bedroom with two other cribs, one on each side of it. The room was generally in semidarkness, for Mrs. Brown was careful of her lights. It was warm—the welfare authorities made sure of that—but only in the afternoon did little Darren see the sun, as it crept along his bed and flickered up against the bedroom wall.

He cried a good deal of the time in the beginning, and he lost weight until Mrs. Brown became alarmed and called the agency. They set up a doctor's appointment then. Mrs. Brown grumbled that she did not have time to go charging off with all these babies to the pediatrician. But she was really a kindly woman, and she knew there was something amiss with this little milk-chocolate colored boy. So one day in the spring she bundled him up and took him to the doctor's office and they sat down to wait in the waiting room.

She waited fifteen minutes and then the doctor saw them. He was grave—the cleft palate and the harelip were the primary problems of the moment. Cleft palate occurs in the partition separating the nasal and oral cavities. It is a congenital fissure in the median line. The harelip is a congenital defect—a cleft in the upper lip. Little Darren was nearly a year old, but could eat only soft foods. He must be kept on such a diet for a long time—until the palate was repaired. The harelip needed surgery too, for him to eat properly.

So there were prescriptions for vitamins and food supplements, and new formulas were ordered and there was a good deal of fuss over Darren. Mrs. Brown complained to the agency that this little boy was taking too much of her time, and that she could not care for him properly. He did not gain the weight that would bring him up to standard, and as he neared two years of age, he continued to look like a baby of one year.

However, despite the inconveniences and discouragement that he brought to her, Darren stayed at Mrs. Brown's for three years. She seemed to grow quite fond of him, and certainly gave him the special care that he needed. He was fed six times a day—milk and chocolate, orange juice, glucose and special vitamin formulas—and slowly he began to gain weight. Mrs. Brown bought him toys when she could, and it was she who took him to get his first false eye.

Darren was late in learning to make noises and words. His harelip made it hard to understand him and he knew—oh how he knew—that he was not like other children. It bothered him. It bothers us all when we first learn that we are different. I've been through it, and I *know*. It's not that we learn we're different, so much, as that we see that funny look that comes into people's eyes. No one is really handicapped. We are all different in more ways than we are the same, and can meet problems ourselves, if we have the will. The will can come from love. It did for me. My mother and father were Italian immigrants, and when I came along, just about half a child with two little twisted stumps for legs, they took my arrival as a challenge to their love. So no matter what else I faced—and I had my problems—I always had my family's love to help me.

Little Darren, he had nothing.

When Darren Dillard was about three years old, Miss Belman, a social worker, came around one day and noticed that he was behind in his development. He was still on baby foods and oatmeal, although his peers were well into chewier fare. She was a bright woman, Miss Belman, and she knew that children can withdraw as well as any adult, thus impeding their ability to learn. She suspected that little Darren was a victim of his environment. She began to think seriously about him. And you could say in a way, that for the first time since he left his mother in the hospital, someone in the world was thinking about a person named Darren Dillard.

Miss Belman carried her work home with her. The image of that slim little brown face, the one side normal, the other drawn up and ugly in its incompletion—the image stayed with her as she went about her rounds. As she visited hospitals and clinics, she talked about Darren Dillard. She learned that the cleft-palate repair could and should be completed now. She learned that the harelip could be corrected in a series of operations so that eventually it would disappear enough so that a mustache would even cover the last scar. As for the eye, and the ear, they were more difficult but could be done. The eye . . . first they had to create a socket, and then an artificial eye could be fitted in. The ear . . . it would mean moving cartilage about and creating an ear. But it could be done. It had been done before. Why could it not be done again? One day Miss Belman took Darren from the house to visit a hospital to see a plastic surgeon. He amplified what she had learned before. In time, said the doctor, Darren could be changed so that the ordinary world would not give him a second look. He need not be a curiosity or a freak. Of course he would never see out of his left eye; there was nothing to be done about this problem. He would never hear out of his left ear. There was no auditory canal, no eardrum. The middle and internal ear were congenitally absent. But all the rest could be corrected, and the boy could be given by man the gifts that nature had denied him.

Miss Belman thought about it. And, with Mrs. Brown's cooperation, she set to work. The first thing she did was arrange for the operation that set up a socket in the left side of his face. An eye was inserted. The socket was not perfect—the eye was out about as much as it was in—but it was a beginning.

From then until 1973, Darren was not given any further corrective plastic surgery. It was somehow forgotten. However, someone was kind to him, for in March of 1972, arrangements were made that brought him into my life. I shall always be grateful for this.

3

The Experiment

What I have said about Darren Dillard in the previous chapters is true, but much of it has been reconstructed over the years since he came to us at Human Resources School. When he came to us, we really knew very little about him. He came with half a dozen others, in a great flurry of confusion, because Darren started out with us as part of an experiment in a particular variety of education.

Before anyone can make very much sense out of my story of Darren Dillard and his new life, we've got to go back more than half a century, to my own childhood. As I said, I was born without legs. My mother told me when I was a boy, "It must have been time for God to send another crippled child into the world. He looked around at all the families. I think He decided that the Viscardis would be a good family to have a little crippled boy."

It is easy to see that whatever I lacked in stature was made up for me in love. My father was a poor man, a barber, and he never got rich. But there was a warmth and wealth in that poor immigrant family living in a New York tenement that I wish every child in the world could share.

When I was little Darren's age, I was in the Hospital for Deformities and Joint Diseases on the upper east side of Manhattan. Most of my early years were spent there, having my poor twisted little stumps of legs straightened out as much as the medical men could do it. So when I talk about Darren Dillard and what was happening to him as a very little child, I know what I am saying. I went through it all, myself.

Actually, although I had no legs, I lived a fairly normal life. Of course I had my troubles. The bullies on the block used to call me "Ape Man". When I first saw little Darren at our school, it came to me that they would probably be calling him names, too, unless we got something done for him. Well, something was done for me and I've been trying to pass it on for the last quarter of a century or so. In fact I was urged to do just this by my old doctor, Dr. Robert R. Yanover, who helped set me up on the artificial legs I now wear.

"There is no bill, Hank," he said when he had accomplished what to me was a miracle. "But someday when you get the chance, do something to help another cripled boy. Then our account will be squared."

I'm still squaring it. And I feel pretty good about the part that Darren Dillard has played in bringing that account to rights.

I know what a handicapped child can do. I proved it for myself once. And just to show that there is no generation gap, I'm watching right now as little Darren proves it all over again.

In my other books I have told my own story, and the story of Abilities Incorporated, and the establishment of Human Resources Center. All this pointed me in a new direction, too, and early in the 1960s we began taking the actions that would lead to the formation of the school.

We knew the need and over the years had accumulated lots of experience. Starting a long time ago good friends began interesting themselves in the problems of the handicapped. Indeed, one of them, Dr. Howard Rusk, renewed my interest in these problems back in the 1940s; he persuaded me to leave a very good job I had, as a personnel director of a large company, and to devote my life to helping others the way Dr. Yanover had helped me. I mention this because we are moving in a new direction these days—toward returning "discards" to the main stream of American life, and one of my important motivations is that I know it can be done. This is very much to the point in the Darren Dillard story.

It is also to the point that by 1961 we had grown to quite a large operation. We owned a large tract of land in the village of Albertson, which is a part of the Long Island town of North Hempstead. Here we had

Abilities, Inc., our workshop that gives productive jobs to handicapped workers, our Human Resources Research Center and Training Institute, which studies the psychological and vocational problems of the handicapped, and a brand new building containing laboratories, conference halls, study room, a special gymnasium where people in wheel chairs can play basketball, and a specially designed swimming pool where people like me without legs, and some much worse off, can swim in safety and comfort. We have since built a brand new planetarium theater.

For at least ten years after we began, I had been thinking of starting a school, and in 1961 we did it. I won't tell about our troubles with the neighbors—some of them—but suffice it to say it was not easy. It has never been easy. Perhaps that is why it is so important to us that it work, and that we accomplish everything we set out to do and a little bit more.

Dick Switzer was with me when we started the school. There could not have been a better fellow for it anywhere than Dick. Like me he is handicapped. He walks with a decided limp and he does not have complete use of one of his arms. He is not *very* handicapped. Unless you saw him walking on the street you might not notice it at all, and while a handicap is an obstacle, in our case, Dick's and mine, it is something of an asset. He and I have no trouble "identifying" with the pupils at our school, and it gives children and parents great confidence to know that they are coming to people who know what physical trouble is all about.

I have told part of Dick's story, too, in the book *The School*—how in the bad old days he was "washed out" of the Industrial Arts division of Oswego State

College because the Dean did not believe that a handicapped person should be teaching industrial arts. Period. It was as simple as that. This treatment, in spite of the fact that he was showing remarkable progress as an education major, working with children in summer programs, that his grades were above reproach, and that he had shown himself able and even proficient in all that he tried to do.

Here was Dick Switzer, over six feet tall and really very little handicapped. Imagine, if you will, what would have happened to Darren Dillard, black, unwanted, with one eye and one ear and that harelip. No matter his brains or charm, he would never have gotten inside the door of Oswego State in 1952. To show how times have changed, it was not so many years ago that Dick Switzer went back to his old college. They were giving him an award for his work at the Human Resources School. They wouldn't let him make a speech though. They *knew* what he might say.

So times change, and they change for the better. By the time Darren is ready for college, with the intelligence he has shown, Oswego State will be glad to have him if he wants to go there. Dick Switzer and a lot of other people have taken care of that.

By the time that I was ready to move on the school, Dick had had plenty of experience in just what we wanted to do. He had spent several years teaching in the Brentwood school district on Long Island, where they gave him the disabled children that could get to school. We were thinking about a much bigger job, but this was fine experience for him.

Our first effort, Dick's and mine, was to plan these brand new facilities at Human Resources Center just as soon as they were ready. We would start with a summer camp. One day I called him on the phone. I didn't dare tell him then that the camp was going to be right next to our workshop. He had to come and see it first, because he was vital to the success of the program. For several years Dick had been taking courses at Syracuse University toward his masters degree in Special Education—which means for the handicapped. I didn't know what he would think of the idea if it came to him cold. So the pool and gym and the trees and the grass that we had brought into our plot were going to sell themselves, with a little help from me. I had already talked this over with Frank Gentile, one of our prime executives in Human Resources Center, and with several others, including Art Nierenberg, the Abilities president, both of them wheel chair-bound.

Dick came on over to Albertson and looked, and liked what he saw. He was out of school for the summer, so we had a chance to start without any dislocations.

Dick wondered where we were going to find the children we wanted for our camp. I was a little queasy about that myself, because we had no idea of how many handicapped children there were in the area. Well, we did not have any trouble getting kids, that's for sure. The Easter Seal Society and the Polio Foundation people found them for us quick as a wink. The minute they learned that the camp was no gimmick, that Human Resources Center was behind it and that it would be operated by Dick Switzer, with his special abilities, they found us a dozen children from eight to sixteen years old—just the kind of spread we wanted

—and half were boys, half were girls.

So we took our first step: we brought these twelve handicapped children to our place for a summer day camp.

Every one of these kids was severely handicapped.

The story of Gil is a good example of the special problems that were posed. He was a victim of spina bifida, a congenital condition in which the bony portion of the spinal canal does not fuse properly and the child's spinal cord is compressed by a cyst filled with cerebro-spinal fluid present at the site of the defect, along with nerve tissue of the spinal cord which does not develop normally. This results in muscle weakness, loss of sensation and absence of bowel and bladder control. The victim's lower body is more or less immobile—the child is usually confined to a wheel chair—and there is the constant problem of incontinence because the nervous system does not control the bladder adequately. The result is dribbling and inadequate emptying of the bladder. Gil had to wear a diaper to control the dribbling. When he wanted to empty his bladder, someone had to rub his belly and press on the bladder area to discharge it.

For all his dozen years, Gil's mother had taken care of him at home. He had never been away from home before, and he had never learned to take care of himself. So while Gil's mother was delighted to have him come to the camp, she insisted that she would have to come too, to take care of him. Remember, these were the formative days. Dick knew that a mother was going to be a drag in more ways than one—camp was supposed to be a *new* experience, and not just an extension of the home. And besides that, Dick Switzer had a few ideas about the handicapped that were much ahead of the times. But he didn't say anything. He just smiled and signed up Gil's mother, and on the first day she and Gil came to camp.

Now, we had a registered nurse at the camp of course, and after Gil's mother had come for three days running, Dick came to me and explained that as lovely a person as this mother was, camp was just not a place for mothers. I agreed, and that day I took Gil's mother aside.

"You know, we have a nurse." I said.

"Yes, I've met her. She is very good and very nice."

"She can do everything for Gil here that you do."

"But I don't want Gil to be a bother."

"He's no bother," I said. "In fact it's a little bit the other way. We want the children to have a new experience alone, and when you are here, some of the other mothers think they should be here too. Really, we can take care of Gil very well. One day he must learn to care for himself."

I brought out all my armament of persuasion, and somewhat doubtfully, Gil's mother agreed to try it out our way for a few days.

What we didn't tell her was that the other children were getting restless, for we had several spina bifida cases in camp, and most of them had already learned how to take care of themselves. We didn't want any regressions on our record.

For the first few days we went according to the book. Either Dick or the nurse got Gil ready for the swimming pool every day. In the locker room they got him out of the wheel chair and changed, and rubbed his tummy and emptied his bladder before he got into his trunks.

Then, one day, Dick decided it was time for action. Gil wheeled himself into the locker room as usual for swimming, and waited. Dick came by and called that he had to do something down at the other end of the building and he would be back in a few minutes. He came down to my office, at the other end, and just waited there. Gil was left alone. He couldn't come out of the locker room until he got his trunks on. And he couldn't do that until he had taken care of himself—or somebody had done it for him.

Always before there had been somebody else. Now he watched as other boys with spina bifida came in, got out of their wheel chairs, accomplished their task, got back in and whizzed out of the locker room to the swimming area, where they could lift themselves onto the ledge and into the pool. Gil was left all alone.

In about five minutes he got the idea. Here he was, stuck in the locker room, and he knew just what to do. So he did it, and when Dick Switzer came back there was Gil in the pool, very busy swimming.

In every way, the summer camp was a great success. Gil's story told us much, for his mother was first astounded and then absolutely delighted to learn that part of the burden she had been carrying for years could at last be lightened. We were sure of it from the beginning, Dick Switzer and I, but like everything else in this business of rehabilitation: "softly, softly, catch the monkey." You go slow and you prove what you know, and pretty soon everyone accepts it without there ever being any argument.

Little Joan gave us another story of proof for our children's program. Joan was ten years old that summer. She was so seriously paralyzed that several doctors had told her mother it was doubtful if she could ever even sit up in a wheel chair. She came to us that summer on a litter. Her new doctors were not even sure she should come; they planned a major operation on one arm, hoping to give her more mobility. But Joan and her parents were so eager to have her enjoy the camp experience that the doctors agreed to postpone the operation until fall.

So Joanie came to us, to join the other cases of polio paraplegia, spina bifida, blood dyscrasia, arthrogryposis, the various malformations of the bodies, arms, legs, hands and feet. From one point of view, a visitor seeing them coming out of their van-buses would regard them as a pitiful lot. But if he waited to shed a tear until he had seen them playing on the special playground equipment we had rigged up for them he might not shed it. And if he saw them in the pool, he would begin to smile. And if he saw them happily engaged in the various games we had designed, he would start to grin. And suddenly he would realize that while it was unfortunate that these kids had to grow up anchored to a wheel chair, they were anything but freaks. And here at the Human Resources camp, they were having a whale of a time for themselves.

Little Joanie certainly blossomed. She seemed to spend most of the summer immersed in the pool. And when fall came, and she was supposed to report to the hospital for the special surgery on her arm, the doctors took a look at her and said they weren't going to do it after all. The swimming had done more than they had hoped to do with the operation.

We came to the end of that summer very pleased with our discoveries and excited about the prospects for the future. It was good that this was the case, because we had no real idea of what we were getting into, trying to change "the system."

4

That Summer

During the six weeks of that summer camp, our dozen children played in the sun, swam, and made leather belts. They even took a boat trip around Manhattan Island, and went on other field trips. And while the kids' dreams were coming true, we were working on our own—Dick and I and other members of the Human Resources staff.

It was our idea that it would be relatively simple to swing from a summer program into school that fall.

As we talked to the children, the need became ever more obvious. For in the early 1960s few, if any, school systems had adequate facilities for the education of the seriously physically handicapped. A building with two or three stories, or just a small number of steps, and no elevator, was out. A building with a basement cafeteria made it impossible. Girls and boys alike needed extra handholds and wide doors in the rest rooms. They could not easily get in and out of buses that were not built for wheelchairs. So the result was that these children, bright as they might be, could have no better than "homebound instruction." Coming back to Darren Dillard for a moment, I must say that although his was a different problem, he and other disabled children in wheel chairs and on crutches were in the same situation. Darren always had perfect use of his arms and legs. His severe facial disfigurement was his basic problem, along with the eye and palate, but so serious in nature that, with the complications of speech and feeding, and the need for repeated remedial surgery, it is unlikely that he would have gone to a regular school. So what I am saying about Gil and Joanie and the others is quite germane to the story of Darren Dillard.

Joanie's mother put it all succinctly one day when she and I were talking:

"They so desperately need education, homebound children. They're like vegetables—they can't move about, but even if you love them they won't change. They need to be in the world around them, with other children, and with someone who cares."

Well we cared. For Joanie had been one of a group of "homebound children." Never again could she be to anyone on our staff. She was Joanie, one of our star swimmers, and we loved her. We wanted to do something for her.

We knew what homebound education meant. In Joanie's case it meant that a substitute teacher from the regular system would try to arrange her schedule so she could come some time during a day for an hour. But many was the day when the teacher would call up and say she had to go to school to take the place of a regular classroom teacher, and instead of coming at nine o'clock in the morning, she would come at six o'clock at night.

"That meant while Joanie was having lessons I was trying to feed the rest of the family. And that was no fun for anyone. It wasn't good for Joan either, because sometimes the teacher would not come for three or four days at a time, and then they would have longer sessions, trying to make up the work. And, of course, there were no extras, like French or music. It was just reading, writing, and arithmetic, and not too much of that."

Three years of that home instruction and Joan was not getting very far although she was a bright child. I could sense, and Dick Switzer told me, that she could blossom under a program of daily classroom instruction. Now it was just a question of bringing it all together.

That's what we thought. Innocents that we were in 1961!

Our first jerk to reality came when members of the staff tried to get figures from the local Long Island school boards and administrators as to what kind of education was being provided for the seriously handicapped in the various schools. The information was not readily available. Several administrators passed us on to staff, to discuss the matter. They were busy with other, more pressing problems. This information was confidential.

I disagreed. I looked down at my own artificial legs and reminded myself that this was very much our concern. There were crippled children in the community not going to school. We were going to find them and bring them to school.

But now I had an inkling of trouble and we were going to be doubly certain to get all our facts and get them correctly laid out. Before fall we had a list of a dozen homebound children who would be available to start our school. We had already been in touch with the New York State Education Department's Bureau for Handicapped Children. We reported to Albany my specific, strong belief that most of these physically handicapped children should be going out into the world to school for the superior education and exposure it would give them. Homebound education with a visiting teacher was not enough.

The school districts of New York State had a well-worked-out program for these children, we were told. They had doctors, psychiatrists, nurses, and educational specialists working with them. They were receiving every attention that education at home could provide. No architectural barriers, no transportation problems; in fact, their doctors and parents all agreed—this was the best system of education for them. So we were told. And with this news, I decided the only thing to do was make a trip to Albany myself. I was confident that with my knowledge and with our camp experience we could "put it over" and secure permission for our school that fall.

Boy, how wrong can you be?

All the way up in my car I speculated on how I was going to "sell" them. Well, I did not sell them anything that day. They listened politely, and they expressed grave reservations that we could possibly offer anything that the public schools did not. They were surprised to hear our objections to the existing school programs of home education. (Nobody had ever raised that point before.) They agreed to investigate further. And that is just as far as we got. There was no committment, no approval, not even a really positive acceptance of my suggestions. I left feeling as frustrated as a person could be. I went home completely down and groggy. Perhaps I had expected too much. It was one of the low points of my career. It took me a good night's sleep before I could even begin to think about fighting the battle.

Next day I called Dick Switzer in. We had been so confident that he was talking about resigning from the Brentwood School District. I caught him in time, and he signed up for another year. I could see the disappointment when I talked to him. Somehow it made me feel as though I had let a friend down.

But I wasn't letting anybody down. We were going to have our school. That was that. It was just going to take a little longer than we had thought.

A few days later things began to break a different way. One of the major officials of the Bureau For the Handicapped in Albany came down and looked over our Human Resources operation, our Research and Training Institute and our workshop. He came to see cripples at work. He saw happy, busy human beings, some of them in wheelchairs, some without limbs, but smiling, working, talking with the vivacity of happy people. He went away visibly impressed. A few days later I had a call advising me to work through the Nassau County Vocational Education and Extension Board, a little-known part of the county government.

One thing led to another, and soon we were back on the track, with plans to open up the school in the fall of 1962. We sent a research assistant around to find crippled children and ascertain their needs and situation. She was the daughter of the doctor who had given me my legs; another part of my repayment program. We put Frank Gentile in as administrator of Human Resources School, and we made definite arrangements with Dick Switzer to come in as headmaster. In the fall of 1961 and in the spring of 1962 we made very careful plans. Dick and I knew now that there could be no slip-ups—it had to be done right the first time.

There were literally dozens of little problems to solve. We secured our permissions, we hired faculty, we established curriculum, and we found our student body and checked into their health problems to be sure they met the criteria we had to establish. We had to be very careful: a child who was coming to the school had to be unable to go to the regular school because of physical disability. He had to be receiving homebound education before we could accept him. We checked family doctors and, if necessary, brought our own doctor to look over our candidates. He was Dr. Leon Greenspan, head of Pediatrics at Dr. Rusk's Institute of Rehabilitation Medicine, and an old friend since the days when I worked with Dr. Rusk for the Air Force, during World War II.

You would be surprised at the things we take for

granted, that Human Resources School could not take for granted. Now my own daughters used to leave the house and get on the school bus at King's Point, where we live. Nobody thought a thing about it. But in our case, transportation to and from the school was an absolute major issue. We had to teach the school-bus people who would provide the transportation, how to fix up van-type vehicles for the use of wheel chairs.

One thing I really wanted and so did Dick Switzer: this was a special school and that much was obvious to everyone, but it was going to be just as much like a regular American public school as we could make it. We had problems, but they were not primarily educational problems. When Dick Switzer went to hire a science teacher, he insisted that he wanted the best *science* teacher he could find. The special problems of teaching the handicapped . . . the new teacher could learn those quickly enough from us if he was interested, and if he was not interested he was not going to come here anyhow, or stay. We had to adapt a lot of things, but we could also remain true to principle: these children were going to have to learn how to adapt to the world, and "difference" was something we wanted very little of.

The kind of problems we met may be interesting; they don't represent difference so much as the adaptation of ordinary standards to meet the needs of the disabled.

For example, we were going to teach typing. All right. Electric typewriters. As any writer or stenographer knows, when you use an electric machine you can get a lot more done in a shorter time, without fatigue. Even the worst crippled of our children should be able to use an electric typewriter. So we went electric.

The classroom. We would start out with 21 students. We would have one big classroom instead of several small ones. Fewer things to get confused and hung up that way. Remember we had a high ratio of teachers and helpers to students, so one classroom did not mean one teacher.

How about coats?

They would hang their coats on racks just like anybody else in any school. The racks just had to be adjusted for wheelchair height.

How about desks?

They would go to desks, just like kids in any public school. Only one thing: the desks would not have shelves underneath. The shelves would get in the way with wheelchairs.

Problems, problems, problems, but such glorious problems, the solution of which would bring these children to life and the love of teachers and fellow students, just like everyone else. It was a pleasure to see Dick Switzer come to work in the morning, smiling and happy, when he showed up in my office at the end of the building. For he was doing something he wanted to do. Every problem solved meant another step gained. Dick was doing something he was proud of. And so was I.

One thing that worked for us all the way was the establishment of our workshop, Abilities, Inc. The people in that office, and out there on the assembly lines were real workers, producing many things for the American economy, electronic devices, computer components for great companies, and even special services for banks and insurance companies. Our children were going to take their lunch into the main Abilities cafeteria. And thus every day they would be surrounded by handicapped people who were out in the world adjusting and producing.

It all fitted in, just like a glove on a hand.

Soon, as we got organized, we had volunteers from the community who would come in and help us meet the physical needs of the children. Dick Switzer, a professional educator, was a little concerned about the use of volunteers.

"What are we possibly going to do with all of them?" he asked me one day.

And out of our experience—we were both handicapped—we began to detail the things that would have to be done, things which would take time: take children to the bathroom, take them to the nurse, mop up spills, write letters for little children, run errands up and down the floors of the building. No, we needed volunteers. It was important for our position in the community that we have them, and it would be important to the volunteers to learn that crippled children are just plain children, with extra problems that love will help solve.

It took a lot of talks between Dick and Frank and myself and many months of really hard work, but finally we had it all put together and the school was ready to open. We ran a camp program that second summer, 1962, and even fielded a friendly visit from Governor Nelson Rockefeller who had heard about us and wanted to see just what we were doing out here on Long Island. We passed the test: he stayed on at least an hour longer than he should have, and had to cancel part of his itinerary that day. The result was that he promised us all the help he could give, and Joseph Carlino, the Speaker of the New York State Assembly, promised the legislature's help, too.

I have told the story of the school in another book, and its place here is simply to make you, my reader, understand what was happening, and Darren Dillard's future once he came to this school. At the time of which I am speaking, Darren was not even born, nor had I the slightest concept that one day we would be bringing in outside waifs. For in the beginning, it was enough to get going, to try to educate and care for home-bound children who came almost uniformly from loving homes. That was our whole concept. Only later did we begin to expand.

From the start, we had big ideas, and we were helped along by our successes.

And we had our problems.

Goodness, did we have them!

One *kind* of problem deserves a little exposition here because it is important to something that happened later at the school; an event that was going to change the life of that little boy who was not yet born, Darren Dillard.

We had specific problems of orientation, even with these children who had been cared for in mostly loving homes. That's not hard to understand if you think about it for a minute.

On that first day of school, Jimmy, one of our spina bifida boys, wheeled himself over to the food line, and took a tray, and got his food and brought it back to the table. He moved in alongside one of his new acquaintances and grinned.

"Oh boy," he said, "That is the first time I ever got a meal for myself in my whole life."

Everything, you see, was new to them. Everything was strange to youngsters who had been in bedrooms and TV rooms all their lives, because nobody knew how to cope with their special problems. And this did not just come to an end overnight.

When we began, there was no precedent for a school of this kind. It was up to us to structure our program into the existing education requirements. The Board of Regents approved our own charter. Of course, we were going to have to work, we knew that, but Dick Switzer and Frank Gentile and I wanted it just that way.

When the word came, we were sitting around in the office and I looked at Frank and he looked at Dick, and we all looked at each other.

"Well" I said. "That is it. Now we've got to perform."

"And there can't be too many mistakes." said Dick.

"There won't be," I said. "I know you too well."

And I did know them and there were not too many mistakes, particularly when you consider this tremendous problem of getting started.

I was talking about orientation. Well, consider it this way: almost all kids past kindergarten age know the street they live on and their last name, and where their house is in relation to the drug store or the grocery store and maybe even the school or the park. But these children of ours did not know where they lived. A street name did not mean anything to them. Even family names meant nothing to some of them. Why should they? Probably nobody had ever asked them these questions before. When confined to a room—no matter how plush a room—it becomes a jail.

So it took a while for us to sort out problems of identity. And then there were problems of success and failure: none of these children had ever competed in games before, so "losing" seemed like a failure and really serious. Or in group games—how could they know what to do when they had never been in groups before? They had to start from scratch to learn how to *play* games, and then how to take victory and defeat —things other children have mastered by the time they hit kindergarten.

I dwell on this a bit because it was going to be a much bigger problem in our school when we finally decided to experiment with resident students—unfortunate children who had no families to take care of them. For if our day students had problems, at least they could go home at night and their families would try to help them sort the problems out. They had the love they needed.

Human Resources School got its charter in 1963. Our next problem was to build a real school building, and we got down to that, too. All we had to do was design a unique school building and raise about a million dollars.

Well, we did. I won't go into that either; it wasn't easy, even though we have a lot of devoted friends. But we managed, and began building up our wonderful school.

Hardly had we begun to accumulate the money when we hit a new snag: our property in Albertson was partially zoned for business, but not for a school.

And when we went before the town zoning board, I was surprised and Dick Switzer was shocked, to see just how many people did not like us. Oh, we had heard some objections before, but we did not realize how many people were upset at the prospect of seeing cripples in the neighborhood. It disturbed their sense of propriety. They had the idea that it brought down the tone of the neighborhood, to have people in wheelchairs, and people with stumps and steel hands moving about. Funny, but there it is. And we have had to live with it.

I hasten to say that by the spring of 1964 the town zoning authorities gave us the variance we needed so we could go ahead with the school.

After that, we started to grow. And we grew, and we grew and we grew. We built our school, and it is a model for disabled people, including those in wheelchairs. I have the feeling that a lot of people not disabled would find some facets of it enticing too—our huge gym, the big light classrooms, the interior greenhouse where the children can see and enjoy plants, and the covered walk that lets them in and out of school in the rain without getting soaked. By 1970 we had a really big school with 176 students, and families from all over Long Island and New York seeking admission.

Unfortunately, the answer was often no. We simply did not have the facilities to take care of all the disabled children who were eligible to come to our school, eligibility being finally determined by the fact that they could not attend a "regular" public school because of physical disability.

Sadly, I must report that we had another quarrel

in our village, before we could build the two-story addition to our school that would bring $3,000,000 worth of construction into Albertson, and put a pleasant new structure on our twenty-acre campus.

More struggle—something I have written about in detail in my book *But Not On Our Block.* This time, our opponents even took us to the Supreme Court. It was costly but we won, and built our addition. I won't try to describe it all right now. I want you to see it as Darren saw it when he came to us, and how this school became an integral part of his life.

For by 1969 we had the idea that not only should we expand our school to take care of as many of the crippled children of Long Island and New York as we could, but that we should establish a residence and bring in waifs. That's how Darren Dillard entered my life.

5
The Residence

One day not long ago, Dick Switzer and Nurse Judy Davidson and I were sitting in my office, which overlooks the front of our campus. It was near the end of a busy day. The late afternoon sun was burnishing up the spring grass, and we were reminiscing a bit about some of our problems of the past.

"Remember when we started the residence" I asked.

Dick's face fell. "That was my fault." he said.

Judy looked at him. "I think it was my fault more than yours."

I couldn't resist a smile. What a pair! "You both know very well that it was my fault more than anybody else's. And as far as that's concerned I'm glad to take the blame even if we made a mistake. Because, for my money, it was about the most successful mistake we ever made."

"It really wasn't a fault at all, you know," said Dick, thoughtfully. "You just have to expect mistakes when you are breaking new ground. Certainly, everybody thought it was going to work."

"And it did," I said, swivelling around in my chair so I could face them both squarely. "If only for one reason, it was worth every bit of the pain."

"What do you mean, Hank?" asked Judy.

"I mean Darren Dillard."

"Oh, yes," she said. "Of course."

"You're absolutely right," said Dick.

And I smiled a happy smile. Because although I am not anywhere near omniscient, in this case it just so happened I *knew* I was right. If it hadn't been for the "mistake", we would never have involved ourselves with Darren.

Foundlings like Darren simply had no place in our program up to the time we opened the residence facility. You can see by now that one of the big problems of caring for the disabled is that no matter how much they learn to do for themselves, they need a lot more attention than any ordinary child. We were not involved with institutions, which had their own various programs for the children. We were involved with some children in foster homes, and in placing some children in foster homes. It's just one of those things we got into because someone asked us.

I think it was the summer of 1970, that it began. Dick Switzer was recruiting students. That always took a lot of time and investigation. For one thing, we had to be sure the home environment was right. For another we had to have real enthusiasm on the part of all concerned—child, parents, foster-parents. Because coming to the school was like going to any school. It meant a discipline and timing, and many disabled children have been badly spoiled and simply cannot adjust to it.

So taking a new student was always a gamble for both of us. If it didn't work out, it would leave a bad taste all around—a thoroughly disappointed and perhaps even embittered child, and a sense of failure among the staff that was hard to wipe away.

Dick was working with St. Agnes Hospital up in White Plains that summer. The hospital had closed its children's unit, and all the disabled children who had been living there had to be moved somewhere. Since we knew a good deal about the families and foster homes all around the Long Island area, we were asked to help out, and so Dick was trying to place some of these children in Nassau County. A real "natural" placement would be to find a family that was already caring for a crippled child of its own. That family would be used to the problems. Quite possibly they could also use the extra money that the community agency would provide for care. And if the personalities worked out, the foundling child would come into a family situation and have a disabled friend to help over the bumps.

This is not so easy to accomplish. People with crippled children are very cautious about whom they take from an institution, and rightly so. Institutions are necessary in our society, but buffeting that comes to little souls in institutional situations creates some strange cases. It was certainly not a question of just numbers—picking up the phone and calling around among our parents and friends to see who might take a child.

Dick was working with Dr. Greenspan, who was familiar with St. Agnes. Also in this group was Miss Lundy, the representative of the Universal Association for Children, which paid the bills for some of these foundlings at St. Agnes.

We had two sets of parents who would welcome another disabled child. When we got involved in dealing with the local authorities and the state, we soon realized that this was time-consuming and exhausting. But we persisted. One family, the Gordons, could not get the license they needed to run a foster home—something to do with the shape or configuration of their house. So there was nothing to be done about that. But we did manage to place one little girl, Susan Feller. She was about twelve years old, a spina bifida case, and she was a darling. They all are in their own ways. Naturally when she came to live with the Barotti family and joined the school we all became very much attached to her.

When it did not work out with the Barottis, she had to be transferred to a county institution. And there was the rub. I have spent enough of my life in hospitals and "institutions" to know how debilitating they can be. They have their special ghetto with all the evils to be found in any slum area. You can get just about anything inside one of these places that you can get outside. And the peer pressures on youngsters, particularly teenagers, are even worse than they are on the outside. Because, remember, for many hours a day, these young people in institutions haven't got anything to do.

We knew *why* the weld between Susan and the Barottis had broken. Poor Susan was already the victim of institutionalization. It's a big word: the connotation is even bigger. A person can get into a rut in an institution that makes him or her actually unfit to live in outside society. Susan, for example, had gotten used to institutional food, and the Barotti's food was different. She had become accustomed to getting up at a certain time, awakened in a certain way. Then she would go to a bathroom and take care of herself. No waiting. No family involvement. She would then have her breakfast, always at the same time; almost always the same food on the same day of the week, week in and week out. She knew what medications she was to have and they came in certain packages. She knew what magazines, what nurses, what the radio and TV rules were—she was used to all this. She had spent nearly all her life in institutions. Nobody cared much, but nobody pried at her. She could not make the adjustment to living with the give and take of family life.

At the school, of course, we had grown so attached to Susan that perhaps we saw her world through rose-colored glasses. Dick and I and Judy and other people talked it over. We certainly hated to put her into that hospital. We knew its reputation. We knew it was a dead-end street as far as ever salvaging the child was concerned.

That was one failure.

It came as quite a shock that same year to see that our second attempt with St. Agnes also failed. This was a boy named John Sommer, who suffered from osteogenesis imperfecta, which meant he had very brittle bones and was likely to break one if it suffered any undue strain. Like Susan, he was a wheelchair student—most of our children are of course. Again for psychological reasons, this placement failed, and still another family placement failed. John eventually might have had to go to an institution.

When Dick Switzer and I talked over these failures, we had an intense feeling of frustration. We had spent a lot of time and effort in that year with each of them and it had been costly. Sure, it wasn't *our* money in the sense of personal funds, but it was money we were in charge of, and we wanted it used properly.

And the money was the least of it. Imagine the emotional investment of Dick and the various teachers and Judy, and some of the students who were friends of these two. No, it was a very unsatisfactory state of affairs, and we wanted to do something about it.

All during this time—and you can scarcely imagine how many meetings and discussions these changes involved—Nurse Judy Davidson and Dr. Greenspan were deeply involved in the whole matter. In a way, Dr. Greenspan was a lot smarter than the rest of us. He kept telling us that these older children who had grown up in institutions were a bad risk in a family situation. And he knew what he was talking about. And because of this, in a way, Dr. Greenspan triggered our idea.

That was the residence plan. It would be a sort of halfway house; not the intimacy of the family situation, which these institutional children resented; but not the cold impersonality of the institutional situation either. They would come to the school, they would live in a dormitory-type arrangement on campus with a housemother and plenty of help, and they would adjust. That was our dream.

When it was verbalized, just about everybody concerned was excited about it. It was a new frontier for us in the care of disabled children, something we had discovered because of our peculiar situation. It seemed to be the obvious way to fill a real need.

I think every one of us involved except Eugene J. Taylor, one of our trustees and a member of our board, thought the residence idea was a good one. Jack opposed it right from the start, although he refused to vote against it if the rest of us wanted to try. He warned that we were getting in way over our heads, and that we were going to end up unhappy. "Disillusioned and sick" is the way he put it. Well as it turned out, Jack was right, and Jack was wrong too. It didn't work, and for all the reasons he said. But I'm not really sorry and I never will be. For even the kids who didn't make it learned a lot from the experience and so did we.

They were fine children. Dr. Greenspan knew more about this particular bunch than anyone. He kept bringing them to the school for lunch, ostensibly so they would have a little outing from the institution, but actually so he could persuade me to speed up our plans to help some of these children.

And of course little Susan and all that she meant to us were very much on our minds all this time, too, because the school year was beginning again, and we knew that what she was missing was going to set her back.

Among several houses on our Human Resources School campus, one was available for a residence. Over a period of years we had bought up the property immediately adjacent to the school, except this one. The man who owned it would not sell in the beginning. But finally, in all the unpleasantness that surrounded our various expansions, we did acquire this ranch-house, and the acreage that went with it. We had five other houses—faculty houses—and we were thinking about moving a faculty member into this house.

Then one day, Dick Switzer was talking to Miss Lundy of the Universal Association for Children about the problem of Susan.

"You know there are a lot of children like Susan under our care," she said.

"It's too bad we can't move them into our orbit," said Dick. "you know we have a house. . . ."

They looked at each other. And then they came to see me.

One attribute I have tried to acquire over the years and which I value highly, is to persevere. That is just about what is needed in situations that involve bureaucracy, eleemosynary institutions, and a new idea.

This difficulty is not the result of human fault but of the unending complexities of social relations in our time.

All that adds up to what I am trying to say. The establishment of our residence meant an enormously complicated set of negotiations, involving government agencies, the Universal Association, lawyers, doctors, architects, and our own specialists. Then there was the question of *What,* and that was as much trouble as *How.* The Association people thought in terms of the foster home. Our ideas were more free-wheeling; we wanted to make the Human Resources School the center of a whole new life for each child.

We finally worked it out; and the Association more or less had its way. It would be responsible for the children during non-school hours. We would approve the children and run the school.

We all felt very strongly and positively about what could be done for these institutionalized children. One day during the discussions, Dr. Greenspan put it very well.

"You know, Hank," he said, "these kids at the hospitals are really in a dead end. The Welfare Department has probably averaged about $60,000 apiece on them now—and as far as I am concerned they might as well have set up a $60,000 trust fund that they could live on for the rest of their lives. That's all the good this system has done."

All that was accomplished, by June. We had our agreement and the lawyers were happy, and we could start moving the children in to take advantage of the summer camp and get acclimated before school started.

First we had to get the architects in and change the house for our children with their special problems. In the bathrooms, the showers had to be modified with special entrances and grab bars that people in wheelchairs need. We have a model shower at the school to teach children and parents what must be done here.

The same is true of toilet facilities.

The modifications did not take that long. Basically it was a problem of adjusting the house to a wheelchair, and literally thousands of American houses are so adjusted these days. Then we were ready to go—to take a housemother and seven children, all chosen by the Universal Association for Children.

That's how I met Darren.

6

Home

The children began coming that Spring to the low green ranch house that we had purchased and for which we now had such big plans.

And we had our disappointments, just as Jack Taylor had warned us.

When the list was set, Dick Switzer came marching into my office one morning with his face all crinkled up, and I knew something was wrong. When Dick isn't smiling, chances are he's unhappy.

He looked at me, and he waved the piece of paper in his hand, and he said, "It's all wrong."

"What's all wrong?"

"The composition. Seven kids, and they go from sixteen down to four."

The four-year-old was fine. I knew that because we had been discussing what we wanted, with the feeling that a big organization like The Association could just wave a wand and supply us with any group in the world.

I looked at the list and I realized we were trapped. For the sixteen-year-old was Susan. All the talking we had done over the past few months . . . if we meant it, we wanted her back. And if we got her back, then we had to accept things as they were, because we *knew* that the younger group would get on better, and we certainly did not want all sixteen-year-olds, with their special "teenage" problems.

When the children started coming in, we forgot about all our worries. Everybody was excited. We met the new housemother, Rose Velez, and were very much impressed to learn that she had once been a nun in a teaching convent. Not only that but she was a biology teacher. Good. We had a substitute teacher right there in the house in case of need.

I did notice that she spoke with a thick accent. Dick learned that she was South American by birth, and that she had not come to this country until she was in her twenties.

But at the time I didn't give it another thought. We were too busy welcoming our new children.

Susan came, and she was all smiles. She had been living at Bird S. Coler Memorial Hospital since she left us. Now in the fall of 1972, she was going to go to Human Resources School once again. We had high hopes for her. And we were delighted to learn that at the hospital she had learned to care for her own needs a great deal better than she had when she lived with the Barottis. One of the problems there had been her inability to cope with personal problems. Now, a teenager, she was reasonably independent, she managed her spina bifida problems as well as anyone we had seen, and the future looked just great for her. She had even gotten braces, and could now walk a bit, although she still spent most of her waking hours in her wheelchair.

We were as pleased to have her back as she was to be there.

Then we met the others.

Paula Murray was fourteen, and confined to a wheelchair as a result of poliomyelitis. She, too, came from Bird S. Coler Hospital. Unlike Susan, however, she had not been out "in the world" for as long as she could remember. She was a purely institutional child. She could not walk, but she was very well able to take care of herself, and she was self-sufficient in many ways. Nurse Judy very quickly noted that Paula kept to herself, although she was friendly with Susan. Even that friendship was quite restrained. Paula liked to crochet. She did many things to keep her hands busy.

The third girl was Nancy Izzo. Poor little Nancy —she had osteogenesis, and her tiny little bones were so brittle that I was afraid to blow on her lest I break one. She came to us from St. Giles Home, which had been almost closed down. In fact, she was just about the only patient there at the end, before she came to us, and she *was* spoiled. They had three nurses there who were assigned to nothing but Nancy. Of course that was temporary. She had not always had three special nurses. But when she came to us that was the kind of treatment she was used to. She could not even sit up, because of her brittle bones, but had to live in a reclining wheel chair. Poor tyke. Her parents had rejected her at birth—they lived somewhere in the New York area—and I am sure she knew.

The oldest of our new boys was Gary Milstone, who was fourteen that year. Like Susan, he suffered from spina bifida, and like her he could use braces to get up for a while, although he was not as active as she was. He was another hospital product, coming to us without really knowing how much he was expected to care for himself. For, in the hospital, someone comes around daily or more often if you are on the schedule, and gives you clean sheets and clean clothes. They change your towels and everything you own. All you have to do is set the soiled things aside, and the hospital personnel takes them off to the laundry.

Of course it was going to be a lot different with us. We simply would not have nurses, and nurses' aides and porters and helpers to be running around picking up laundry and changing things when it was not really necessary. We were going to have to teach our crowd a lot of self-care. Why not? When they grew up, most of them, at least, should be able to care for themselves and cope with the problems of life in a wheelchair. As our home-raised children have almost all learned, that's part of life. And most of them want to take care of themselves. It is a matter of pride.

And, of course, we could not afford the kind of laundry service that is used in a hospital, nor was it necessary. We installed an automatic washer and dryer in the house. Those two appliances should take care of our new "family."

The second boy in terms of age was Michael Hirten, who suffered severely from congenital limb deformities—so severely that his family, *decided they simply could not cope with Michael's problems* and turned him over to New York's welfare services. It was not that they were uncaring people, or unthinking. But they had several children, Mrs. Hirten worked very hard to keep them neat and clean, and Michael demanded an effort she did not feel she could make. His legs end above the knees, which meant that the attachment of a prosthetic device was most difficult. He had no forearms—only stumps.

Yet in several ways Michael was the most normal of our children. Occasionally he went home for a visit, usually at such times as Thanksgiving and Christmas. Apparently these were not always happy experiences. One time when he was home he realized that his mother was shielding him—keeping him away from the window, and when someone came to call, swiftly wheeling him into another room so he would not be seen. That knowledge was not very helpful. In some ways Michael must have been glad to be back at the residence after such a visit, and back at school, where his difficulties do not even attract attention, for everyone is used to them.

Michael had another advantage. He had been under care in Dr. Rusk's Institute for a long time, and he had prosthetic legs. But with his little stumps they were difficult and the boy did not like to use them, and so spent more of his time in the wheelchair than he should have. In fact he spent most of his time in his wheelchair.

I am not being hypercritical. I know what that is all about. It takes a tremendous will and a tremendous drive for a man without legs—and particularly without knees—to manage artificial limbs. You spend a lot of time flat on your face on the floor, after you have lost your balance. Anyone who doubts this should feel my upper arm and shoulder development. The one compensation is that I have shoulders and upper arms that are about twice as well developed as the average man's.

They didn't get that way automatically. But Michael had no upper arms, only stumps to break his fall, or to hold on with to prevent a fall. Walking on artificial limbs would always be difficult. Mastering them was not impossible—others had done it. But he had long since given up, and no longer really cared to try. He would spend the rest of his life in a wheelchair.

Michael had a lot of problems. We were not aware of all of them when he came, and it probably would not have made much difference to us anyway. Using his stumps, he was probably the fastest and most versatile wheelchair operator in school, and he also could play a fair game of basketball. He was a big boy, and because of his lack of limbs perhaps, his trunk was highly developed for his years. He looked older than his thirteen years. And one thing we noticed right away. He got along very well with the smaller children. That was going to be a real plus.

The sixth of our new children was Todd Hansen, the next-to-youngest. He was six years old that year. Todd suffered from a cardiac weakness, stomach problems, and some congenital deficiencies. He had a cleft palate, and he showed some indications of DiLang Syndrome—small muscles, thick eyebrows, and tilted-up lip and facial weaknesses.

In almost every case the physical problems of the children have a good deal to do with their behavior patterns. It would seem mean, for example, to say that Nancy cried a lot and whined for what she wanted, unless you knew that it was a symptom of her condition and completely to be expected. It is remarkable, when you have a few such facts, how quickly you are able to adjust and pay no attention to the expectable problem that might otherwise annoy you.

Todd had very real and immediate problems that would have to be dealt with. His cleft palate and weak stomach meant that he had difficulty eating solid foods. He also suffered from serious psychiatric problems. For some time little Todd had lived with his mother, and while this can be wonderful, in his case it was not. There had obviously been some real difficulties and for weeks after he came to us he would wake up crying. He also suffered from insomnia, which in a child of six is a terrible problem.

And then, finally, we got Darren Dillard. He was the baby of the crowd, only four and a half years old when he came to us.

In a way, he was the least handicapped of all. He had full use of his arms and legs and no cardiac impairment, so he could run and jump and play. He did have only one eye, and a very badly done socket that let the false eye fall out when he moved suddenly. He had no hearing in the left side of his head, still no semblance of a left ear, and the bone structure on the left side of his face had not completely formed. As he grew, because of the flattening of his face, the left side sank in, and the appearance of severe facial disfigurement became more marked rather than less so.

So they came in, one by one, and the staff clustered around Susan in her wheelchair, waving and smiling and shouting "Mr. Switzer—Dr. Viscardi—hi —hi—I'm back!" And Paula, her chum from the hospital, following close behind in her wheelchair, and little Nancy coming in by ambulance, and the two bigger boys, and then little Todd, who also came by ambulance although he was not confined. And finally, by car, came this little black boy, in a gray shirt and short black pants. He got out of the car with Miss Lundy, and held back between her legs, dragging and yet smiling very shyly.

I had gone over to the residence on my electric scooter that afternoon. That's how I usually get around the campus because while I can walk, its not that easy to cover nearly half a mile from one end of the campus to the other on a pair of artificial legs.

I was standing there, passing the time of day with Miss Velez, the housemother, and Nurse Judy and Dick Switzer, when suddenly out from behind Miss Lundy's skirts stepped this skinny, disfigured little boy about thirty inches tall. He wrapped his arms around one of my legs, and looked up shyly.

"Hello," he said. "I like you."

I looked down at him. Here he was, a little boy who represented precisely what we hoped to achieve —just over four years old, with the world laid out before him, ready to be conquered. We had the tools, and we would teach him how to use them, and then one day he was going to be ready to go out into the outside world and face normal American life.

It was a thrill to me, I'll tell you that.

7

Stefanie

I said in the beginning that this is a story of love, but I did not tell what I meant specifically, or whom. Now I shall say that the real beauty of this tale lies in the love that developed between this half-blind, half-deaf little black boy in our Human Resources School, and a bright and attractive girl in her late teens. The boy, of course, is Darren Dillard. The girl is Stefanie Kaley, elder sister of one of our Human Resources students, who was a counselor in our summer day camp, and who is presently the research assistant to Dr. Marie Meier, of Human Resources School.

To understand how and why Darren came into Stefanie's life and assumed a big place there, you first have to know something about this pretty girl and her family. Then you can begin to understand.

Stefanie was born in Flatbush in the heart of Brooklyn, into a hard working middle-class Jewish family. Before Stefanie's mother and father were married, her mother lived with her parents, Mr. and Mrs. Dorsky in a big red brick apartment house. After Lou Kaley came along and married Roslyn Dorsky, the young Kaleys moved in with her parents because the Dorskys needed them. The Dorskys, husband and wife, ran a lunchroom-restaurant down in the middle of Manhattan's garment district, and for 38 years the two of them got up at 4:30 in the morning and went to the restaurant. Five days a week they did not come home until eight o'clock at night. Only on weekends did they live a "normal" kind of life. So they needed the Kaleys to help take care of the big apartment. It was a mutual undertaking—real charity on both sides. It worked very well, and the Dorskys and the Kaleys always lived together, even after the children came.

Stefanie was the first. She was born in 1952 in a hospital not too far from the apartment house. That red brick building became her home, and she grew up learning to ride up and down in elevators and play in the parks. Brooklyn was a quieter place in those days and Stefanie saw no trouble. She started kindergarten at P.S. 217 and went straight on through with good grades and with the smiles of her teachers. She went on to Ditmas Junior High and then to Midwood High School. Like many other children in a middle class family, her life was centered around the home. Her playmates came to the apartment, and she went to their apartments to play and to sleep over, as teen-aged girls love to do.

When Stefanie was four years old, another little girl was born to the family, Alisa. She was sick from the moment she was born. The Kaleys had to leave Alisa in the hospital for a week. During the first three years of her life, she had to see many doctors and spend numerous weeks in the hospital.

When Alisa was three years old, the medical men announced gravely that she was suffering from dysautonomia, a disease of the autonomic nervous system and very difficult to manage.

Alisa does not have tears. She suffers from diminished tear production and has to be given artificial teardrops. She has no sense of pain. She could cut her finger on a toy and never know it. She suffers from motor incoordination and has very diminished reflexes.

One day Mrs. Kaley became very upset because Alisa vomited her milk, and just kept on vomiting in what the doctor diagnosed as a cyclic attack. These cyclic vomiting attacks are another symptom of dysautonomia.

As she grew older, she seemed to fall behind. When she tried to walk, sometimes she grew dizzy and faint, and had to lie down. Sometimes her blood pressure would spurt up, and that would make her dizzy. It would then drop, which also made her dizzy. Sometimes she had trouble breathing, and had to use a respirator.

Little Stefanie watched gravely as her mother worried over Sister Alisa. She ran to the night table to get the eye drops. She ran to the bathroom to bring out medication when it was needed. She tried to help, and as she helped, she grew to understand that Alisa was not quite like other children. She was sick. Because of Alisa's illness, Stefanie was given much responsibility, causing her to mature at an earlier age than most children.

Sometimes Stefanie would come across her mother sitting over a cup of coffee at the kitchen table, silent. She knew it had something to do with Alisa.

And in those days there seemed to be a lot to think about. Because fifteen and twenty years ago the prognosis for children with Dysautonomia was a short and uncomfortable life. It has changed now, Thank God and medical science. But it used to be said that such children could not expect to reach sixteen years of age.

The Kaleys were first aghast, and then sad, and maybe a little grim, and then a great peaceful understanding settled over them. They were not a tremendously religious Jewish family—that is they did not keep a Kosher home, but they did celebrate Chanukah and Passover and other religious holidays. Their culture, more than their religion, was Jewish. The walls were hung with religious art. They had love to spare —love for Stefanie, love for each other, love for relatives, and a lot of love left to devote to little Alisa, as long as she might be with them.

Mr. Kaley, an optician in business, decided that he could best serve his daughter's interest by working with parents of other children who had this same disease. So he joined the national organization of dysautonomia and eventually became one of its vice presidents. The members were dedicated to helping each other, to passing on information, and to doing everything possible to strengthen their ailing children and bring length and joy to their lives.

As long as Alisa was with the Kaleys, she was going to have the best care that they could afford and find for her.

That is how the Kaleys first became involved with Human Resources School. They learned of our school through Sylvia Levinson, whose daughter also had dysautonomia and attended our school. At the time there was no way we could get together, because they were living in Brooklyn. One of the school's hard and fast rules—we have to be that way—is that the school districts that want to send their handicapped children to us *must* provide the transportation. Brooklyn was too far. So while Stefanie went to neighborhood public schools, Alisa went to a public school in Brooklyn too, that had a class for children with physical disabilities.

It was a problem, as everyone in the family knew and understood. For in this particular class there were nine children with various disabilities, in four grades —from first to fourth. There was only one teacher in the classroom, who was responsible for all the material in the four grades.

"She didn't learn much in that school," said Stefanie sadly, when she thought about those years. "There were too many levels represented in the one class, not enough room, and too much going on all at once. We could tell she was getting behind."

The more Lou and Roz Kaley considered the problem, the more they felt that they must find a place

for Alisa to go to school where she could be given a
real chance. It was not long before Mr. Kaley was
visiting Human Resources School. And as Stefanie
approached her graduation from Midwood High
School, Lou and Roz Kaley knew what they had to do.

They were going to buy a house on Long Island,
in an area where they could be sure that Alisa would
be able to attend Human Resources School.

Graduation day came in the spring of 1969, and
Stefanie lined up with 1300 others in cap and gown to
receive her diploma and hear the charge of the com-
mencement speaker to those who were going out to
face the world. Her parents were there with her. By
this time, the Dorskys had retired after those 38 back-
breaking years of running the restaurant. Grandfather Dorsky was pleased with the idea of having a
little plot of ground, and Grandmother Dorsky liked
the idea of a house.

As for Stefanie, her thoughts were elsewhere.
She had just won a partial scholarship to Hofstra University, and when the speaker talked about the great
wide world, she knew what she wanted to do. Her
sister's illness had sharpened Stefanie's eyes to the
needs of the world; she would go into the kind of work
where she could help people like Alisa and some who
were even worse off in so many ways. For all that was
wrong with Alisa was physical. She had a good mind,
and a patient family—and a household full of love.

Watching people in the streets and in her school,
Stefanie had seen how rare were these commodities,
and she knew that her goal in life was going to be to
bring care and affection to some of the world's ill-
treated. She would become a psychologist, and she

would major in psychology in college.

Of all those concerned with the coming move, Lou Kaley bore the greatest burden. For years he had been connected with a large New York optical house and had risen to a managerial position in one of the Manhattan offices. It was true that his firm had expanded to Long Island, and maintained a number of shops in various communities. But who could tell—if he moved out to Long Island and asked for a transfer from his present office, he might set himself back on the economic ladder. It was a chance he had to consider. There was also the risk that Stefanie's scholarship would not be renewed after the first year. What would she do then? Mr. Kaley could not afford to send Stefanie to Hofstra on his own. Having considered all of the factors known to him, he decided that the overall welfare of his family came first. He would move.

For Mrs. Kaley, it would be a wrench as well. For years she had busied herself with her group of friends. They enjoyed each other's company and worked closely in an organization devoted to charity work. But she did not even need to look at Alisa, and the glow that came into that girl's eyes when she considered that she would be going to Human Resources School. Mrs. Kaley had no trouble deciding to make the move.

The house hunt began.

Every Sunday the Kaleys scoured the communities of Long Island for the right house, and they found it on a quiet residential street in Syosset. It was a pleasant, middle-class split-level house of a design much favored by Long Island builders in the late 1950s. There was plenty of room for the family, and a flat yard around the house where they could grow flowers and even a few vegetables if they wished to experiment in the sandy soil.

Then came moving!

What a job. The accumulation of twenty years had to be unearthed and sorted and either packed away or discarded.

And then the day.

The van came up, and Alisa clapped her hands at the excitement. The furniture kept going out, until the good old apartment looked like a dingy cave. A hasty look about in the suddenly unfamiliar territory, the comfortable confusion of getting the family down and into the cars to take them to the new house, and then Lou Kaley closed the door of the apartment behind him, and went to enter the new world they had chosen.

Alisa came to camp that summer, and was both delighted and delightful. She fit in immediately. She swam in the pool, and played on the swings and moved about in our very own boat, specially constructed for disabled children. We had picnics and hot dogs, and trips into the field, and managed, in our buses, a trip to the shore, and many other excursions that summer. But best of all, the children said, were the activities we put together right in our own back yard.

As with most of our children, the camp, and then later the school, became the most important part of Alisa's life. She felt at home here. And why shouldn't she? For the people around her—the other disabled children and adults, and the non-disabled—are all people "who understand"—people with sympathy and no long stares for someone "different." Here she saw Alex, who has been working at abilities since 1952 and, who gets about all over the acres of campus on his half stumps for arms and legs—a man who is invariably courteous and smiling *and* productive, in spite of being about as badly handicapped as anyone could be.

And of course as Alisa slipped smoothly into the routine of camp and school life, Stefanie watched and marveled at the changes in her sister. Alisa seemed to grow taller. Not one of her dangers was minimized: she still might choke to death some night, or her respiration might slow and even stop; those were the dangers of her disease.

But at school and at home, Alisa smiled more, she perked up and had more interest in life around her. Like some others facing the drab future that she saw before her back in the bad old Brooklyn days, she had slowed down. It was not unusual: many a *handicapped child* gives superficial evidence of being retarded. But no more of that for Alisa.

And as they talked about it all at home, the Kaleys could smile at each other in that secret way of happy families. They all knew that they had made the right decision.

8

Stefanie and Darren

During her years at the school Alisa blossomed brightly. Stefanie, who was pursuing her course in psychology, found herself drawn more and more to the school, and what spare time she could muster was spent in helping out, particularly in the summers. In her second summer she was again a Camp counsellor. She did so well at it with her quiet, sympathetic manner and her firm good humor that that year we made her Head Counsellor. That was the year that Darren came to us.

Four-year-olds have a charm all their own, and

Darren was no exception. He had just acquired the complete mobility of a four-year-old, and he had the agility of a gazelle and the stamina of an elephant. He was on his feet, up to something, all the time. For a little while, it seemed that Darren might even be hyperactive. The housemother said so. That was quite a mystery, for his medical record showed no such complication. And then, we had reports that he was retarded. With so small a boy that would be a little harder to gauge. But we still did not believe it. In a few weeks the real trouble raised its head: it was the housemother and not any of the children. Rose Velez simply was totally unsuited for the job.

We got into it because of Darren. She complained that he was noisy and disobedient, but volunteers who came to the residence said they did not think so and at nursery school, Mrs. Steinberg, the very experienced nursery teacher, said she saw no signs of waywardness. So we investigated. Poor Miss Velez—or should I call her Sister because of her nun's background? That was the trouble. She had never been married, she had never realized until she came to us that all children are a lot of trouble. She expected adult behavior, and instead of that she had children who by family standards were dreadfully spoiled. The older ones—those who had been in institutions for a long time—complained if dinner was not served exactly at 5:30. That's when they had been used to eating. And as everybody knows, once someone gets on that kind of schedule, the stomach growls by itself. And the children from hospitals did not clean up after themselves. So Miss Velez had her complaints, too—the washing machine was running all day long, she had to rinse and clean dirty garments by hand before they could be washed; she was chasing all over the house, cleaning bathrooms and picking up. She was overwhelmed by the job, and it *was* a big one.

Poor Miss Velez. I felt sorry for her, but very much relieved to learn from Nurse Judy and others that Darren was not the problem. He was the *victim*. He liked to help, so he tried to pick up things and carry them for her. Sometimes he made a mess. Then his harelip did not help much. He had spent so much time alone and in incommunicative circumstances that he was hardly articulate when he came to us. Imagine—Miss Velez, who had difficulty with English anyhow, trying to get along with a small, very unsophisticated black boy born with a harelip!

Your imagination will tell the rest.

Miss Velez had to go.

That decision created a problem, not within the school, but in our own structure. The Universal Association for Children was not pleased, but realized we had a situation that needed to be changed. By mutual forbearance, we managed to secure the appointment of a more suitable person. At least we hoped so. Now, in hindsight, I can see that we were much too cavalier in our approach to the housemother problem. The other day I was talking to Dick Switzer about it, and I said just that.

"That's not quite true, Hank," he said, "Because you forget that we were not really in control."

"I did forget that," I said. "Then *that* was our mistake."

"You're being very tough on us," he said. "Remember, the Universal Association would not do it at all unless they could run the housing, and we didn't want to do that because we were not equipped to do it."

"Well, next time. . . ."

That conversation reminded me just how much we *were* feeling our way, back in 1971 and 1972. Really, as Dick says, no one is to be blamed, but if we were to do it again it would be done quite differently.

Perhaps this explains a bit of what happened in the housemother department in the few months after Miss Velez left.

Next came a pretty young nurse from down south someplace. She lasted for a few days, and then quit. She should never have tried it, she said. It was too big a task for her physically. She went on home.

So we got Ellen Lawson. Now she was the best of the lot. But in this time of troubles, we had also spoken around Human Resources of the need for some help at the residence, and that is how Stefanie got involved over there too—as a volunteer.

I think Stefanie was about the first outsider to do so. And when she did, she encountered Darren.

She went over to the residence one day, after her classes at Hofstra had ended, and checked in to see what she could do. The dishwasher was empty, and the sink was full. So she settled in the kitchen to do some dishes.

In came Darren, as hungry a four-year-old as you have ever seen.

"Whatcha doing?" he said, "I'm Darren. Who're you? Whatchagotoeat? Where's Ellen? Let me help."

All this was announced in one blast, and by the time Stefanie had a chance to speak, Darren was already climbing up on a chair to help put glasses in the top of the dishwasher.

She began to field the questions one at a time.

"I'm Stefanie," she said, formally. "Glad to meet you."

"What does glad to meet you mean?"

And at that moment, Stefanie's heart went out to this little waif that nobody wanted. She knew he was for her.

So there were cookies and milk, and there was some more washing to be done, and Darren ran the vacuum in the living room, while Stefanie dusted. By the time the dusting was over, and the vacuum cleaner put away, they were fast friends.

Two or three times a week after that, Stefanie would come to the school or to the residence. She had no responsibility as far as her sister Alisa was concerned at the school. That was our job. From the time the kids were picked up in the morning by their own district bus driver, until the time they were delivered back home in the afternoon, they were ours, so when Stefanie came to the school she came to do other things than take care of Alisa—who was much too busy anyhow with her own affairs to spend a lot of time with Big Sister.

But Darren was the magnet.

A month after she began coming, they got into a conversation about shopping.

"What's shopping?" he asked.

"You know, you go to the supermarket and buy cookies and milk."

"What's a supermarket? he asked, very serious.

Stefanie caught a sob that was starting in her

throat. She had not realized, until this moment, what a wall existed around this little boy and the other children who had been sloughed off into professional foster homes and institutions.

"Would you take me to a supermarket?"

"When?"

"Right now?"

Stefanie looked at the clock. It was four in the afternoon, and she did not have to be back for supper for an hour and a half. Nor would the children eat dinner until later.

"Let's ask Ellen."

So she asked, and approval was granted with a smile. Off they went, then, in the car that Stefanie shared with her mother, since Hofstra was an impossible walk and there were no buses from the Syosset house.

A few blocks from the school was the local shopping center complete with A&P, drug store, cleaner—all the stores that Americans are used to finding in these malls. She parked the car. Darren struggled a little bit with the door handle, and she watched, smiling, but did not help. Suddenly it gave, the door opened, he nearly fell out, caught himself, and gave her a big grin. She grinned back and did not help him get out or close it.

Hand in hand they walked into the A&P, Darren gazing around in astonishment first at the row of red plastic and shiny steel carts outside, in their straggly nest. He marveled at the automatic door that opened when Stefanie wheeled the cart onto the rubber treadle, and he ducked behind her and slipped out the "Out" door—to try the "In" door once again, coming up behind the bewildered girl.

"That's neat," he said. "Do all stores have those?"

She explained that supermarkets were not like other stores because people came and bought lots of groceries for a whole week and had to have a cart to carry them out to the car.

"You mean they let you take the cart with you?"

"To the car."

"Don't they think you'll steal it? Some kid stole my racing car one time. In the hospital."

"No, they don't think we'll steal it. It's what they call the honor system."

"What's that?"

Stefanie was sorry she had ever mentioned the honor system—but he was pointing at the long white case where the cheese and butter and eggs and milk were kept. It extended along almost half the store.

She explained that case then, as he stared. And she showed him the meat cases, and the canned vegetables, and the long counter filled with crackers and breads and cakes and cookies. He selected a package of Oreo cookies to take home with him. Stefanie took him to the candy counter and bought some gum and candy bars for all the children at the residence.

"You mean all this candy's here to take? I'll betcha somebody steals a lot."

And then it was time for a little lecture on the honor system of supermarkets, after all. She delivered the lecture, and Darren listened.

"Then I won't never steal nothing from supermarkets, I promise."

"Won't ever."

Won't ever what?"

She laughed. That was the end of the first lesson.

9

Home Life

The first time that Darren came to the Kaleys' split-level house on its curving drive, what impressed him most was the flowers. It was summer, the roses were climbing along the rail fences, and a dozen other plants were sending out blooms of red and pink and blue and purple.

"Look at all the flowers," said Darren, pointing out the window of Stefanie's car, as they drove into the Kaley driveway. "I never saw so many. What are they?"

So before they could go in the house, Stefanie had

to take Darren on a tour of the garden. He fingered the roses, and Stefanie taught him how you could squeeze off a rose petal, crush it between your fingers, and make perfume. So there was nothing to be done that afternoon but to make perfume for Todd and Susan and Paula and all the rest. They went down in the basement, found half a dozen old jars with lids, and spent the daylight hours mixing up perfume to take back to the residence.

"Don't forget Ellen," said Darren gravely as they bottled up and counted. "She would get a thrill."

Stefanie looked at the small black boy and began to laugh. "What?"

"Get a thrill. You know. A good feeling."

"Where did you learn that word?"

"I heard Mrs. Steinberg say that last week when she came in with the bumblebee in the jar. She told Ellen she thought our class would get a thrill out of seeing a bumblebee."

There was nothing to be done, then, but to go out and pick more roses, and crush them with the rolling pin, and put them in a jar half full of cold water and shake them until Darren was quite sure the perfume would be strong enough to impress even the nursery school teacher.

Until the perfume was made, Darren had little time to talk to Roz Kaley and by the time the last bottle was capped, Lou Kaley had come home from his office. He was the gardener. He spent another half hour outside, explaining to Darren how plants grew, and when they came in the little boy was full of new-found knowledge.

"We saw an apus," he announced at the dinner table. "He nearly bit us."

Lou Kaley laughed. "An aphus, not an apus, Darren. And he didn't nearly bite us, I sprayed him so he would not eat the flowers."

"All right," grinned Darren. "He was an aphus. Anyhow we saw him. And if we were flowers he would have bitten us."

Everyone laughed. It was a pleasant dinner.

There were many such, that summer. Stefanie spent her days supervising campers at the school, and as a resident Darren was automatically a camper. She saw him every day, and watched him blossom as did her father's roses, in the newfound friendship and attention he enjoyed in the residence. It was not an institution, but of course you could not get away from the fact that the residence was not a real home, and the housemother was not a real mother or big sister to them. It came to Stefanie most clearly on those weekends when she took Darren out. Wasn't it too bad that she could not help little Nancy and Susan and the others? What they all needed was love. In watching, Stefanie saw clearly that enough love could cure the most dreadful ills of these children, for the worst hurts were not their physical difficulties, but the wounds inflicted by society. The secret was to *care*. And she cared, and the awful loneliness and hurt eyes of the children made her want to cry.

One day Stefanie came into the residence to help Ellen Lawson with the sandwiches they would take out on a picnic.

Darren, of course, was helping. Ellen was supervising the making of tuna fish sandwiches, and Darren's job was to open the refrigerator and get out lettuce and mayonnaise and whatever else she asked for.

He could not find the mayonnaise.

"It's right there," she said. "Right in front of you. Can't you see?"

Darren stopped and turned his head from right to left inside the refrigerator, and then he found the mayonnaise, tucked over in the left-hand corner.

"I'm sorry, Ellen," he said. "It was on my bad side."

Ellen Lawson stopped, pursed her lips and said nothing. Stefanie began to cry. It would have taken so little for Ellen to have touched Darren, to have apologized for her show of bad temper. And the look on the little boy's face was worst of all—for Stefanie could see that Darren blamed his inefficiency on his disfigurement. She could sense that he was telling himself, "Well—I'm a cripple and of course I'll get yelled at."

So Stefanie, tears clouding her eyes, grasped Darren to her, and hugged him, and hurried him out into the sunshine where they both could have a new look at the life around them.

"That wasn't your eye," she said. "That was just carelessness."

"You really think so?"

"Of course. People drive cars and they can even pilot airplanes with only one eye."

"Boy, that's what I'll do."

"Drive a car?"

"Anybody can do that. Be a pilot."

And he spent the rest of the afternoon zooming around the playground, arms outspread, being an airplane. The mayonnaise was forgotten. The hurt erased by love.

As the summer passed, Stefanie could sense that

some of what she was doing was destroyed each day by Darren's encounters with others. For the children in the residence had varied experiences; about the only thing one could say was that they all came from institutional situations, and they reacted in that way. The love that Stefanie could give was assessed and diminished every night. When Darren brought home his perfume, Michael poured his bottle down the toilet. "Perfume is for sissies," he said. Nancy put hers on the shelf and did not even smell it. Susan smelled hers and said it was too weak to use. And Darren of course, was disappointed. He told Stefanie of the reaction of the others.

"That's just the way brothers and sisters would act," she said.

"No they wouldn't. These kids are just jealous 'cause they didn't get to make it."

And of course Stefanie could see the logic, the constant competition among them for approval of the "normal" people in the world outside. When she and Darren were alone, when Darren came to her house, he was a different boy. And remembering, she could see the changes—see how it came in waves—how Darren would relax and learn at her house, and how the push back into the residence where "they did not understand" was like being thrown back into the fishpond.

Ellen Lawson tried, but there was too much to be done for her to maintain the emotional reserves necessary to create what we had planned—a home situation. Instead, the residence was a halfway house. Certainly it was better than an institutional life; every one of the children improved socially in some way. Darren showed the greatest improvement of all, because of his youth, perhaps, because of his greater mobility, perhaps, but mostly because of that indefinable—the love that was transmitted almost every day from Stefanie Kaley and from the Human Resources School.

There were others who came to the residence. Luckily, they showed that different partiality of human nature for different types. Caroline Schanck, a camp counselor I remember, was a volunteer who helped Ellen Lawson that summer. She would come in in the mornings and do dishes and clean the floors and start the never-ending operation of the washing machine and dryer. She was friendly and got on well with all the children, and she learned something that not one of us in administration then suspected—that we were sitting on a tinder box.

The real problem was the older children. Susan and Paula soon found they disliked their life for it was not working out at all the way they had hoped. They were used to living in the hospital—and before they came back to the school they had been going to a public school.

"I hate it," Susan told Caroline one day.

"Why?"

"Because my friends are all at Bird S. Coler and here I am, stuck here."

And then there was the special problem of Michael, who was Darren's hero for a while. He taught Darren to play basketball, and it didn't make any difference that Michael was in a wheelchair—knew the game. But Michael, poor Michael—he could not learn to read. He was too old. Here he was, a teenager, stuffed into class with little kids who outshone him every day. He was 13 and could not even read a comic book. He knew some letters and a few simple words, but could not read.

And as it was with Stefanie, so it was with her friend Caroline Schanck, another girl with all the love a heart could hold.

One day I was talking with Caroline about the situation in the residence.

"What about Michael?" I asked.

"There's something hard about him that I don't understand," she said.

"You mean he's mean to the others?"

"He isn't. It's just when somebody from outside tries to get at him . . . I can't reach him. I just feel he needs love, and he wants it desperately, but if you do something nice for him, half the time he will reject you."

"How?"

"Well, one day I thought I would do something for all the kids so I brought them each a candy bar. Michael took his and bit into it and spat it out on the floor and threw the rest down. And then I had to clean up the mess."

Such a story was not too uncommon. Children are little human beings, but they can become dreadfully twisted and confused by life even before they reach puberty. And I could sense that in our residence we faced problems that we had never faced before, because we had never before tried to manage children on a twenty-four-hour basis.

We were, of course, facing the total needs of the handicapped, and we were becoming a little dismayed about resources and our present ability as a school to bring these children what they really needed.

In this atmosphere, day after day I saw Stefanie and Darren together, and there was no mistaking the pleasure each found in the company of the other. I did not totally understand but I contented myself with watching. Whatever was happening there was obviously for the best. Darren, who had come to us as a frightened little rabbit, was now all over the place.

Darren and Todd Hansen shared a room at the residence, and they were friends, or at least friends in the way that a six-year-old and four-and-a-half-year-old could be. Todd's big problem as far as daily life was concerned was none of his outward physical deficiencies, but his hyperactivity. He was nervous and constantly in motion, from waking in the morning, until the light was out and the housemother had checked on him for the last time.

We understood that he was on tranquilizers, and that they helped pull him down toward normality, but his level of activity was still very high. Darren was so bright and so responsive, however, that Todd did not seem to upset him in the way that another might have been troubled.

Big Michael was good to them, too. He spent hours in the gym playing games; on the playground he would be sure they were in his group. And they were proud and stuck together with Michael. Gary, the other boy at the residence was older and much more advanced, and so quite outside this little group.

In the afternoons they assembled before the television set to watch the children's programs. It was like a ritual, five days each week. And on Saturday there was a *whole morning* of shows to delight them.

When Darren and Stefanie went out together they talked about life in the residence.

"It's not like your house," said Darren. "Everybody fights."

And that *was* a problem. The children, being children, were sometimes fractious and upset as they faced new circumstances. Being crippled exacerbated their troubles, certainly. What we had not really allowed for was the necessity of a very close ratio of "normal" people to meet far more than the physical needs of these young people. We were doing well. We could see progress. We did not estimate properly the dryness of the tinder; but perhaps it was beyond us to do so. Only later did we begin to understand the tensions more fully.

The summer of 1972 passed pleasantly, and by its end, Darren was more than ready for kindergarten. It might not have been so—his emotional development might have instructed that he stay on with younger children. But his own innate brightness, and Stefanie's love and attention brought him up several notches in a hurry. By school's starting time Mrs. Steinberg, the nursery school and kindergarten teacher, and Dick Switzer were marvelling at Darren's vocabulary. We knew, of course, that vocabulary was related to people, and Dick observed that this was obviously Stefanie's doing, not ours.

So it was a happy and well-adjusted boy who started school that fall, the happiest of the children in the residence, leading a busy life, exposed to the processes of learning, surrounded by friends and sympathetic people, and moving about tentatively in an outside world that most of his young friends in the residence neither could see nor wanted to see.

Summer became autumn, and fall then passed. Stefanie was busy with college, and the days of summer when she spent the waking hours mostly at the school and camp were long behind her. Yet Stefanie did not forget Darren, nor he her, and almost every weekend Darren either went for an excursion with his college friend, or she brought him to the Kaley house to spend the night. One day they went to the big green park, a few blocks from the Kaley house, and Darren had his first taste of the outside world of children— one he had never really before entered.

Stefanie was wise enough, when she saw the small boys playing marbles, to stand back and see what Darren would do.

He held her hand for a while and watched. When one boy shot his marble too hard and it chased across the dirt into the grass, Darren dropped Stefanie's hand and ran after it, marvelled at its beauty and carefully took it back to the other boy who waved a flippant thank you. Then he stood behind that boy, having staked his claim, and when one of the boys got up guiltily and said he had to go home, the boy with the marble offered to teach Darren to play. Stefanie retired to a bench and watched from afar, as Darren Dillard entered the real world of "normal" children without a tremor. Only once did she see anything worth noting. Half an hour passed, and Darren completed with flying colors his first lesson in "migs." She spoke to him on the way home.

"I saw that boy point to your face," she said.

"Oh yeah."

"What did he say?"

"He asked me what was wrong with my eye, and I told him it was false. He thought that was pretty neat."

In some company, Stefanie might have gasped. In still other company, she might have laughed. But she did neither. She nodded wisely as if it was totally normal to expect people to behave with compassion and wisdom, and for six-year-olds to do it too. So Darren, that fall, was living in the best of all possible worlds for him.

10

The Dog

November came with its blowing leaves, and the
ground turned chill. There was football in the street
and in the park near Stefanie's house, but that was
only on those weekends when Darren was taken
"home," and then only for a few precious minutes it
seemed. For Stefanie could not simply turn Darren
out of doors at the house and let him make his own
way as he would have done had he been her own. She
was too unsure—she not he—for already in fewer than
half a dozen encounters, Darren had established himself in the community of the little kids of the park as

more than a stranger. He didn't go to their school, and
he wasn't around all the time so he couldn't be a regular. But he was certainly accepted.

"Do they ever ask you about anything?" Mr. Kaley said at dinner one night.

Darren knew what was meant. He was direct.

"You mean my ear and my eye and stuff?"

"Yes."

"No."

"You mean nobody ever asks you?"

"One kid did—I told Stefanie. Nobody else did.
They can see I haven't got any ear."

Lou Kaley, too, marvelled at the resilience and
tolerance of the young. And he was wise enough then,
to see beyond his own eyes, too. So Darren's hold on
the Kaley family increased as the months wore on and
he became a welcome, if irregular, visitor to the family
table and the family hearth.

And the change came in other ways. With Gary
Milstone and Michael Hirten, Darren clustered
around the television set on Saturday afternoons and
Sundays. The girls fluttered away to do needlework or
take care of other chores, and little Todd roamed the
house, getting into things in the kitchen, or nervously
wandering. But the three other boys were glued to the
television. Football. And of the three, only Darren
could play—he had played in a wobbly scrimmage
over in Syosset—and he would play. He dreamed of a
football helmet and shoulder pads and a jersey and real
football pants.

Stefanie observed the growing interest. And one
day she asked Darren. She was greeted by a question.

"You think I could catch a pass with one eye like
those guys do on TV?"

"I don't know why not. I think so."

"That would be good. You see them run. I can run like that. And the helmet would hide my ear."

So he was still sensitive about the ear. And why should he not be? He was moving ever toward the general society. But what Darren did not know, and those around us like Dr. Greenspan did know, was that Darren could have an ear and would have one. For as we moved in one area, the Universal Association and the New York authorities moved in another. Darren was going to be made whole by society's standards, if it could be done. His once cleft palate was filling in nicely. His harelip needed one more operation, and then a few years for scar tissue to subside. He was on his way in a lot of directions, and not the least of them was his precocity, which had developed only since he had gotten to know the Kaleys so well and had been exposed to love.

That's how it was as the calendar pages turned to November. It was cold, although we had not yet had our first flurry of snow that announces the arrival of old man winter. It was cold and foggy on Long Island.

By the time school ended in the afternoon, and the children from the residence cleaned up and ran their errands down to the office and watched their friends get off on the buses, it was growing dusk. Todd and Darren and Michael, the triumvirate of the residence, fooled around a little bit in the gym with the basketballs, if there was someone to watch them a little late. Otherwise they went on back to the house, and watched television until time to clean up for dinner.

Everybody ate, according to his or her habits. Some of them were finicky, and subsisted mostly on bread and butter and milk, it seemed. Some, like Michael, ate so much you wondered how they packed it all in. Darren ate well as a rule—mostly soft foods, because he had trouble chewing. But little Todd Hansen did not eat well. With his cleft palate, he was unable to chew and swallow anything the slightest bit tough, and his stomach problems made digestion difficult. Todd would turn from tough foods to milk and juice—not very happily, because, as he grew, he had learned to like the taste of meat.

Dinner over, the children helped by taking their own plates to the sink (those who could manage) and they gave Ellen a hand with scraping and running errands around the kitchen and putting away food. Darren was always helpful; the incident of the mayonnaise was long forgotten.

Shortly after supper Dick Switzer would "happen" in for a quick visit. It was not a "happening" at all, but a careful part of a plan. For the last few weeks, warned by Carolyn, we knew that the girls in particular were not happy, that the residence was in danger of falling apart. So Dick and Nurse Judy Davidson made a point of dropping in once a day just to check. It was not hard. Dick lived about seventy-five yards from the house on another street, and Judy lived in another faculty house about the same distance away.

The girls then gossiped and the boys watched TV. Soon it would be time to turn it off—before the violence of prime time began.

In the matter of TV, we were particularly careful about Todd Hansen. Not long before, we had learned that he had psychiatric problems we had never considered. If we had known about them, probably Dr.

Greenspan would not have recommended his inclusion in the "family." But now that we had him, we were trying to work as best we could. He liked to stay up late—he suffered from insomnia and slept very badly. But the programs of violence were dangerous to his weak heart and the exaggerated conflicts did nothing for his psychiatric troubles either. So the television was policed as rigidly as we could manage.

But with Todd we were either too little or too late. For November was not finished before Barbara Steinberg and Dick Switzer came into my office one afternoon with very long faces.

I looked up.

"Who?" I asked. Not what but who. For I knew only a problem regarding one of the children would occasion so much worry.

Barbara flashed me a brief smile. Dick looked embarassed—that look he gets when he thinks he has failed.

"Todd Hansen. Barbara has got to suspend him."

I looked at her. She nodded.

"It's the fifth time this month, Hank. The whole kindergarten is a chaos. He won't stay in his seat, he won't do what he's told, and now he has taken to temper tantrums. I'm afraid for the safety of some of the others. You know we have three osteo. . . ."

She needed to say no more. Osteogenesis—one of our greatest problems, for the young children have bones that break on the slightest impact. They simply could not be left at the mercy of a hyperactive child who was not under control.

"Have you talked to Judy?" Of course they would have. But I asked anyhow.

They nodded. "He's getting all the tranquilizers the doctor will let him have. He's just out of control."

"Would a temporary suspension do it?"

Barbara was thoughtful. "I doubt it. I've put him out for a day at a time. Poor kid. He doesn't want to be ugly. He just can't help himself. But he's dangerous . . . . . ."

"All right," I said, and I must admit to my reluctance. "Suspend him. But let's think about it for a week or two. If there's some way. . . ."

They nodded glumly, and filed out, as mournful a pair as had trodden our long halls in many a month.

I long ago learned to take a firm stand in life, and I remember when others would have thrown me out as a misfit, so I made the judgment that Todd was to be kept around the place a little longer. Out of school, he really had no place with us. We were not a "home" for the handicapped—the residence was strictly a part of the school situation. But I know that I was most reluctant to declare any failure, and I am sure that Dick Switzer let things go too, because secretly he agreed with me.

So Todd was taken out of school, but kept in the residence. It was not fair to Ellen Lawson; it made more work for her and I am not sure we compensated by giving her two more volunteers to help look after the children. But what I did not expect, was the story of the dog.

Someone in the neighborhood had given us a puppy. He was not dog-show material, just a short, fat, brown, cuddly puppy of no particular breed. Only by looking at his paws could we estimate that at some future date he would be of watchdog stature. At this moment the puppy, whose name was Wags, was a bundle of brown eyes, wet tongue, and love.

Among all the children, he took to Todd most, and after the second night began sleeping on Todd's bed. Darren was a little bit jealous. Sometimes he could persuade Todd to let Wags sleep in his bed for part of the night, but always during the night sometime Wags would disappear from Darren's bed and next morning he would be found in Todd's. Darren was a sound sleeper. He did not wake up when the dog was taken away.

One night about a week after the suspension, Todd was more restless than usual. He quarreled with Darren over their toys, which was odd but not totally unusual. He yelled when he was given his evening tranquilizers, and tried to hit Ellen. And that night after lights were out, and the boys were in bed in their room, with the door closed for the night, from Todd's bed, Darren could hear thudding sounds and the sharp cries of the puppy.

"Whatcha doing. Hitting the dog?"

The sounds stopped.

"He was bad," said Todd. "He peed on me."

"Want I should get Ellen?"

"No. It wasn't much. It'll be all right."

So they settled down again to sleep. Darren was hard to wake, but during the night he woke up because he thought he heard noises and crying. But when he was awake and listening, there was nothing. Soon he drifted back off to sleep.

Morning came, and with his usual smile at the day, Darren bounced out of bed, and ran into the bathroom to be the first to brush his teeth. He brushed mightily, and combed his hair in the mirror and washed his brown face. Then he headed back to the room and got out clean underclothes and a clean shirt from the dresser. Clean socks, and yesterday's corduroy trousers—they should last two or three days, depending on the mud. And he put on his clothes and did everything but tie his shoes—because he was not yet good at knots.

While he was dressing, Todd Hansen was getting up. Out of the corner of his eye, Darren could see Todd get out of the bed and throw the covers back up. He caught a glimpse of something brown. Todd dashed out the door before he could be questioned, and into the bathroom. Darren stood up, and instead of heading for Ellen in the kitchen, he looked under the covers of Todd's bed. Then he ran.

Ellen Lawson came. Nobody remembered to tie Darren's shoes for another half an hour. For when she came to the bedroom and looked under the covers, there was the puppy, dead and cold.

They brought Todd, and he began shuffling around the way he did when he was about to go into a spell of hysteria. Michael had come in, and Paula and Susan, and they all just looked at Todd.

"Why did you do it?" cried Susan, and she began to sob.

"Because he peed on me. And then he tried to bite me," said Todd furiously. He moved to the bed and began striking down at the little corpse. "Because he was bad, he was bad, he was bad!"

II

The Fire

The next turn in the story, you might say, was either the whim of fate, or my carelessness at being out of town at the wrong time. I *think* that I should have recognized the need to take swift action on the morning that the puppy was killed. But because I had been so reluctant to move Todd out of our ambience altogether, Dick Switzer and the rest simply suffered in silence and waited for me to come home and make the decision.

By the time I got home the excitement had quieted down, and although I heard of it, the telling was almost incidental—there was always so much going at the school that an event a week old seemed like ancient history. So, not being warned by worry or tone of voice in the telling, as I certainly should have been on the day the puppy was killed, I put the matter aside with a frown, hoping against hope that something would come up to alter the inevitable decision to ask the Universal Association for Children to move the boy somewhere else.

There were other signs of trouble. But the problem is that you never know them all. When you are dealing with children you are lucky if you know half of them. And when you are dealing with children and changing staff as we did so often at the residence, then it becomes most difficult indeed. *Two years later,* I learned that in the summer when the children were keeping rabbits and kittens at the residence, a kitten was left alone with Todd Hansen, and it died under mysterious circumstances. Had I known that in December, 1972, plus the story of the dog, I most certainly would have acted with celerity.

Then came an important evening in the first week of December. They were having Swiss steak for dinner at the residence. That is an odd factor in the story, for if they had not had Swiss steak and it had not been tough, then things might have turned out another way. By this time, except for the troubles of Todd, the residence was really shaping up quite well. The three girls had adjusted, and the two older ones took marvelous care of poor Nancy, our Miss Brittle Bones. There were games and many parties—always birthday parties and affairs to celebrate any kind of holiday. Even cleanup was made a celebration of sorts, and there were often little rewards of candy or a favor for a job well done.

But the Swiss steak was tough, and Todd Hansen could not eat it. So with reluctance, he went back to his diet of cottage cheese and milk and bread and butter and liquid supplement that did not bother his cleft palate, nor his weak stomach. He was upset and angry most of the evening, and particularly after Michael teased him because of his bad behavior. Todd grew very red in the face and dashed off to his bedroom and hid under the covers.

After the incident of the dog, Ellen Lawson had taken Todd into her room to sleep, so that she could keep an eye on him. But tonight he ran into his old bedroom, and when Ellen came to look for him at bedtime, he either was asleep or pretended to be, so she went away and left him in his bed.

When bedtime came, Darren went to his room as cheerfully as usual. He undressed, got into his pyjamas, brushed his teeth and washed his face, and got into bed, and ten minutes after Ellen turned off the light he was sound asleep.

Sometime later—it was dark and the house was all quiet—Darren was awakened.

"Hey, Darren," came an urgent whisper from beside his pillow. He opened his eye. It was Todd.

"What do you want? Go to sleep. It's night."

"Can't sleep. Wanna smoke. Do you wanna smoke?"

"Smoke what?"

"Smoke a cigarette. I've got two. Found them in Ellen's room."

"Go ahead. Smoke. I'm sleepy."

"Haven't got matches."

"Then go to sleep."

"Come on," said Todd, tugging on Darren's pyjama top. "Let's get matches."

"Go away," said Darren.

But soon the tugging was so insistent, that to avoid the irritation and to keep his pyjamas from being torn, he sat up in bed, rubbing his eyes—for he kept the plastic eye in his socket unless it irritated him.

"What do you want?"

"Get me matches."

"You know where they are, in the cupboard."

"Can't climb up."

"You can climb up just as well as I can."

"Can't."

Darren knew very well that the older boy had climbed up into the cupboard before, but he also knew that Todd was afraid of the dark.

"You'll start a fire," he warned, as they headed for the kitchen.

"Won't. Wanna smoke."

"I'll tell," said Darren, suddenly afraid that Todd really was going to start a fire.

"You tell and I'll sock you," said Todd fiercely, grasping Darren's arm.

They had come to blows before. Todd, with his bad heart and all was still three inches taller and a good ten pounds heavier than Darren, and could overpower him in a struggle. So Darren went along, and they sneaked in the dark into the kitchen. Todd got a chair from next to the refrigerator, and put it up against the counter on the side where the matches were kept. Darren climbed up, opened the cupboard with one loud squeak, and scrabbled around with his fingers until he found the box of kitchen matches that was kept up there to light the gas stove if the pilot light failed. He took out a handful of matches, grasped them firmly, and swung down to the chair and then to the floor.

"Give them to me."

"What are you going to do with them?"

"I'm gonna smoke. Wanna?"

"No, I'm going to sleep."

Quietly, they crept back to their room, and Darren got into bed, while Todd stayed outside his bed and sat down on the floor at the foot of it.

Soon, Darren was disturbed by the smell of sulphur.

"What are you doing? You're lighting a lot of matches."

"Gonna smoke," said Todd. "Gonna smoke." And he laughed a laugh that Darren knew meant hysteria. There had been plenty of that before.

Darren jumped out of bed, and grabbed the matches off the floor. They wrestled, and Todd took a swipe at Darren with his arm, hitting him in his good eye, and knocking him back.

"Gonna smoke," he said. "You stay away from here."

By this time the smell of smoke was evident in the room, and looking over at Todd's bed, Darren could see that the wooden bedstead was on fire and blazing. The covers caught and began to make more smoke and soon both boys were coughing.

Darren headed for the door to warn the others, but Todd, eyes wild with panic, stopped him before he could get to the door and they struggled. Just then, the elaborate smoke alarm system that had been installed when the house was converted began to go off, and the alarm shot off its warning signal.

"Fire," shouted Ellen Lawson, and she ran to the rooms to be sure that all the children were awake and could be gotten out.

Out of his room sped Todd, with Darren trailing behind.

And then out of the house across the street stepped Dick Switzer. He was opening the door to let the cat out, and his next move would be to yawn, stretch, and go to the kitchen to start the coffee for breakfast.

Just then, as he let out the cat, through the mist he smelled the smoke and heard the sirens ringing in the residence.

And he knew—the residence was burning.

12

The Firebug's Trail

When Dick Switzer peered out of his doorway that morning and saw the smoke coming from the residence one thought rushed through his mind:

"My God, the kids are gone."

For he knew that most of them could not manage in an emergency. A flashing fire, coming through a bedroom where Nancy or Susan were sleeping would get to them before they could ever scramble out of bed and into their wheelchairs. If the fire had raged, then indeed the children were gone.

But as Dick stood there, the Albertson Fire Department arrived. Seeing, he dashed back into the house, stripped off pyjamas and dressed and then rushed to the residence.

Judy Davidson, the nurse who lived next door to Dick, had almost precisely the same experience and the same reaction. By the time the two of them reached the house, Judy in her housecoat, the situation was under control.

Rushing through the house, Todd and Darren had awakened Ellen, and she had moved swiftly. First she had gone to the room where little Nancy slept, picked her out of bed and taken her out to her car, and put her in the seat where she would be safe. Then she had returned to be sure that the less crippled children were dressing and getting out, even as the fire spread from the boys' bedroom.

Soon all were evacuated, and the fire department was in charge, moving hoses and spraying the house and nearby homes to prevent spread of the blaze.

"Damned good thing you had that system," muttered the chief to Andy Panzarra, the school's chief of maintenance.

And of course, the chief was right. Here was one time our care had paid off, even more thoroughly than we expected. For our fire system was connected directly with the Albertson Fire Department communications. It not only warned of fire, but went into action when smoke began to accumulate. And when the fire had begun in the boys' room, the intense smoke created by the burning mattress had triggered the alarms before the wood really caught. So the fire department had what we might call advance warning. Five minutes after the alarm went off, the department was in action and on the scene. The children were clustered about the front of the house, and the residence was blazing, with gouts of fire and smoke coming out of the kitchen and the bedrooms.

By this time I had been called. Dick had seen that all the children were safe, and then, sleepily, half in shock, had gone back home to notify me. There occurred then, one of those early morning conversations that in retrospect tend to break you up because they are so inane:

Scene:

Viscardi bedroom. Henry Viscardi sound asleep. Time: 6:30 A.M.—one half-hour of blessed sleep time before getting up. Condition: cold, foggy, dark.

The telephone rings. Viscardi fumbles and picks it up sleepily.

"Hello."

"Goodmorning Hank I have some bad news the residence is on fire the children are all right."

Silence. Then—"I'll be right over. I guess you had better be excused from our weekly breakfast meeting this morning, Dick."

So then I got up and got dressed, and went to the scene.

It was all under control. By that time, Dick had six of the children in the school cafeteria which is warm and bright, and they were having breakfast. Poor Nancy had suffered a broken bone while sitting in Miss Lawson's car, and she was on her way to the hospital for treatment.

But there were problems. The fire had been extremely destructive. It had burned through the roof. Nearly every room had suffered damage. The flames had burned so hot they had fused the electric motor of the refrigerator in the kitchen. In the boys' room everything had been destroyed and in the other rooms wheelchairs and prosthetic devices were lying on the floor half burned away.

An immediate problem: all the children's belongings were gone. They were in their nightclothes, every one of them, and nightclothes were all they had left in the world.

In times like these, you see the benefits of organization. Years before we had established our Human Resources Center Auxiliary and the members of that volunteer force had been smart enough to set up emergency procedures which we now realized would be useful for just such a matter as a fire. Dick Switzer got on the phone, and in a matter of minutes the switchboard was in operation and calls were going out in all directions. The need was clothes for the seven children. Before noon we had so many clothes for them that every child was as well off as before, and some of the excess had to go to the Salvation Army.

All the children were dressed, then, and all but Nancy and Todd Hansen were sent to classes as the other children arrived around ten o'clock. Todd was no longer in school, and Nancy was at the hospital. So Todd stayed under Judy's guidance that morning, while I checked to be sure that Nancy was getting the best possible treatment and that there were no complications. There were none. Broken bones for osteogenesis children were a common occurrence. Nancy had had many before. For her it was a way of life.

Earlier, I had told Dick Switzer he would not have to attend the weekly staff meeting that morning.

Well, neither did I. For as I sat in the cafeteria, drinking a cup of coffee and listening to the excited accounts of the fire and rescue, it suddenly occurred to me that my troubles and those of the school were only beginning. Immediately we had to find some way of taking care of seven children who were homeless and frightened. They were excited and busy right now, the centers of attention, but in a few hours all this would wear off, and the reaction would set in. Whatever else we had accomplished in a few months with the residence, we had at least established a functioning home for seven children, and now it was so badly wrecked that it would be months before normal operation could be resumed.

Dick's day and mine were spent in finding housing for the children. We went down to my office where I sat behind the desk and Dick sank into one of the leather chairs, and we considered the matter. Slowly, as the day wore on, we sorted out the children and matched them up with volunteer parents.

Gary Milstone, the teenage boy, was no trouble at all. He went to the house of the Huysmans, a family we knew. We knew from the beginning that it would work out fine.

Michael, the big boy who could not read and had no arms below the elbow, was a more difficult problem. He was something of a bully, and that meant we ought not to force him into a situation where his negative qualities would create trouble. So we solved that by putting him into a family with an older child. That was going to work all right as well.

Susan and Paula were no real problem on a short-term basis. They were well-behaved girls. They would have liked to be together, but they could recognize, with the perspicacity of all our children, what a burden that would be to any family. So they parted cheerfully enough, and went in different directions that afternoon as the buses came.

Nancy, I discovered in mid-morning, had a small fracture of a thigh bone. The doctor was very cheerful about it—it was a crack, not a full break, and ought to respond very nicely to treatment. But we were not going to have to worry about Nancy for a couple of weeks.

So there were the problems of Darren and Todd to be resolved. And that presented us with some serious considerations.

On the lawn in front of the burning house, Albertson Fire Chief Douglas Diem had raised the first question.

"How do you think it happened?" he asked Dick and Miss Lawson.

And that started us all to thinking, even though in the early hours of the morning other matters pressed.

We had spent thousands of dollars to be careful. We *knew* we were careful. We doubted if anything could be wrong with that expensive and well checked wiring, or with the new heating system. The fire had started in the opposite end of the house from Miss Lawson's room so there was no question that she might be smoking in bed, or otherwise careless.

At the end of the morning, when the smoke was cleared away, and the firemen were clearing out the debris, Dick and I left the office and went over to the house with Chief Diem.

"How did it start?" The question was in all our

minds. And until it was settled, we could not make any positive decisions about the future. Indeed, we were holding back a little on deciding just what should be done with Todd and Darren, because the dreadful suspicion had already entered our minds that they might have set this fire. On the lawn, Ellen Lawson was quick to see that those two were out before her—and so wide awake that they seemed to have been up for some time. A quick suspicion flashed through her mind—she had noticed that the fire was hottest in the end of the house where the boys slept. But it might have started in the kitchen, too.

So we went into the house. What a shambles. Every piece of furniture was burned or charred. Not one could be used again. The overstuffed furniture was burned, and smelled of smoke, and was dank with water. All the appliances in the kitchen were ruined, the cupboards were burned and even the food inside was charred and had run into a sticky mess.

In the bedrooms the dressers were burned, and the clothing inside destroyed by fire or smoke. In Michael's room, his artificial legs had been burned, and they lay there on the floor, black ugly reminders of the tragedy.

We wandered around the room, shocked at the destruction and wondering how long it would take to repair. Chief Diem was looking for something, but we were not so skilled as to know what. Then, when officials of the Nassau County Fire Marshal's office arrived, the chief and the experts searched further. When they were finished they gave us their opinion. Somebody was probably playing with matches in the boys' room.

It was just what we feared. For that morning

people had begun to remember things. Miss Lawson had remembered that Todd and Darren were caught playing with matches one day. Caroline Schanck had corrected her: Todd was playing with matches and Darren was trying to get them away from him.

Or was he?

That afternoon we conducted our own investigation. We had to do so—it would not be fair to send these boys off to friendly homes and a few nights later learn that they had burned the house down. Very carefully, we approached the problem. Dick worked at one end and I at the other.

In midafternoon, Dick came in to me and said he had discovered that Todd Hansen had been playing with matches several times before, that Darren's part in it seemed to be only incidental, at worst, and that there was some indication that Darren had tried to stop the older boy from this dangerous play.

The thing to do, then, was to go to the source. And so we got Darren to go to the nurse's office. That way—for he was in and out cleaning up the eye and repairing scratches—there would be no "big deal" that would frighten him or make him feel that he was under surveillance.

Dick sat in. I did not. It would have been too much.

Darren came in, and Dick and Judy began to ask him about the fire.

"Tell us about the excitement."

"I was asleep," said Darren, "and then Todd started lighting matches. That woke me up."

"What did you do then?"

"I got out of bed."

"Did you talk to Todd?"

"Yep."

"What did you say?"

"Whatcha doing?"

"What did he say?"

"He said he was smoking. Not to tell or he'd sock me."

"And then?"

"I tried to take the matches. He socked me. And then the bed was on fire. We ran."

Dick looked at Judy and Judy looked at Dick.

Just to be sure, they went to the gym, where Todd was playing by himself, and they asked him about the fire.

"I dunno," he said.

"Did you have any matches?"

"No, not me."

"Do you know how the fire started?"

"No."

"Were you asleep in bed?"

"Yes, I was asleep."

"How did you wake up?"

"Darren woke me up."

"Were you really fast asleep?"

"Yes I was."

And that, of course, was the tipoff. Because Todd, of all the children in the house, was the only one completely dressed. He had gone to sleep in his bed earlier, or pretended sleep. With his history of insomnia, it was quite obvious that he woke up in the middle of the night. For since he was "asleep" at bedtime, he had not taken his usual tranquilizers. And then he must have awakened in the early hours. Much,

much later we learned from Darren that Todd had pushed him into getting down the matches. This was not the day for that kind of questioning. But we had our answer, certain enough to make a decision.

Darren was innocent enough. Todd was our firebug.

13

Crisis

Now Dick Switzer and I had to make one of those hateful decisions that confront people in authority from time to time. We had to take action that would have vital effect on the life of another person.

First we got Judy to do some of the dirty work. We had her call Bellevue Hospital in New York City to secure admission for Todd Hansen. Or to try. Our rationale was simple; Bellevue has one of the most effective psychiatric systems of all the hospitals in the area, and it is big enough—a teaching hospital—to care for all of Todd's many problems. As for school, he was already out of our school. This latest escapade made it impossible to try to rationalize his return under any conditions. So Bellevue was the proper place for him, from our point of view.

But not from Bellevue's.

"Six years old. . . . cardiac condition. . . . cleft palate. . . . Not for Bellevue. . . . try one of the children's hospitals. . . .

"They will not take him. He has psychiatric problems."

"Sorry. . . . try another. . . ."

So I got on the phone and argued, to little more avail. Then we got Dr. Greenspan, and he argued, with no more success.

Only when we did what we did not want to do, and laid the fire strictly at Todd's feet, could we get him admitted: we had to tell Bellevue that it was almost certain that this boy had set the fire that destroyed the residence and endangered the life of all those people. Then Bellevue agreed to take Todd Hansen.

It was with real self-hatred and pity that we let him go, knowing that whatever had prompted this six-year-old to his play, he had not seriously been trying to murder anyone, or even to destroy the residence. It was an accident; playing with matches was obviously an attention-getting device—and we had cast the boy to the lions. He was going to a psychiatric hospital now with a record. His life would never again be the same.

But we could not think that way. We had hundreds of other children to consider, and immediately the six others who had been uprooted by the fire.

By late afternoon, all were settled but Darren. We still had the problem. He *had* been involved. We were morally certain that his involvement had been minor and under coercion. That was all we really wanted to know, although for some time the nagging doubt would persist. But, having taken appropriate action, we could now proceed to place Darren somewhere.

I knew where. There was no doubt about it. He would go to Stefanie Kaley and her family, if they would have him. Of all these "placements" for a few days, this was by far the most natural, and with the burden of the fire off our backs, we set about getting in touch with Stefanie and her parents.

It was raining heavily that day. The morning had been consumed with the details of the children's welfare, and the afternoon with the problems of the fire. So it was late when we got around to finding Darren his place with the Kaleys. Mrs. Kaley was actually not at home, but at the office where she worked part time. The Dorskys, Mrs. Kaley's parents, did not drive often and both spent most of their time at the house, so Darren would have no shortage of companionship. But how to get him "home." Alisa, the younger daughter, who attended our school, had already left on her bus, so that was no good. Dick and I worried about the problem—it is a twenty minute ride to Syosset from the school. But then in came Stefanie, fresh from classes at Hofstra, braving the pouring rain and gray skies, to come and get her friend.

What a sight.

Here was Stefanie in her tan trenchcoat, dripping from the brim of her hat to the bottoms of her galoshes, standing in our gym and shaking her umbrella. There was Darren, dressed in a huge shirt and a pair of oversize trousers that belonged to Dick Switzer's ten-year-old son, held up by a piece of rope. But at least his sneakers fit him, and he was moving around the gym floor as if nothing, not anything at all, had happened to him that day.

And when he saw Stefanie, he dropped the basketball and rushed across the floor.

"Hi, Steffie," he shouted from across the room. "Guess what?"

Stefanie always played the game.

"I don't know. What?"

"We had a fire. That's what. Oh, boy, was I scared. But you know what else?"

"No."

"Well, I was in my pyjamas. And we all had to run outside. And I didn't get pneumonia."

So he rushed up to her, and wet coat and all, he snuggled against her, the little black boy with one eye and one ear, standing pressed against the handsome girl, pretty even in the bedraggled state of a rainy day. I wish I had had a camera.

But I can say that again and again, for there is the story of love between these two, the white Jewish girl and the little black Protestant boy—so natural that it is hard to believe without photographic evidence. It is the story of what might be in all America and all the world when we are as near perfect as those two. It is a story I see before me every day and one that never ceases to delight me. Loving is to love that which is unlovable or appears to be—then it is vital.

Stefanie and her family on the one hand, and

little Darren on the other, are walking testimonials to human love. It existed between Stefanie and Darren long before the fire, of course. I have no way of really knowing how the Kaleys and the Dorskys felt about the little black boy when Stefanie brought him home for this stay. I have the feeling that the Dorskys' adjustment might have been the most difficult: they were old country people, Russian Jews who had never encountered a black before they came to America. And yet being of the persecuted, their transition may not have been so hard.

So they went home that afternoon in the pouring rain, and Darren told Stefanie, the Dorskys, and Mrs. Kaley all about the excitement at the school and all about the fire, while they waited for Lou Kaley to come home.

Lou Kaley is a practical man, a neat dresser himself, a student of clothes, and when he came home that evening from work, the first thing he noticed was Darren's ragged costume.

"Come on," he said not five minutes after he had entered the house.

"Where?" asked Darren. He knew Mr. Kaley well enough to ask that kind of question.

"To the mall. We're going to get you some clothes."

Stefanie suggested that she and her mother take Darren shopping. Mr. Kaley agreed.

They drove to Jericho turnpike, and to the mall, and they began searching. It *was* a search. From one shop to another they trudged, trying to find blue jeans (oh, how Darren wanted blue jeans) and corduroy trousers for a very small boy with almost no hips and bottom at all. And shirts and underwear, and new sneakers and a pair of good shoes. And he needed a couple of sweaters, and a jacket. Everything was come by the hard way, trying on and trying on, until Mrs. Kaley and Stefanie were wondering how small boys lived in a world built three sizes too large. But finally it was done, and Darren went home with them, fingering his parcels, looking at his new shoes, and quite at peace with the brand new world the fire had brought him.

It was "only for two or three days" I had said to the Kaleys and to all those involved with the children who had been victims of the fire.

How wrong can one be? It was two or three days before we even had the insurance adjustors out to examine damage, and then endless complications arose because of the nature of the fire. Until that was established, the premises had to be left alone. If there was criminality involved, which there might have been in the eyes of the law, then the evidence was not to be inadvertently destroyed.

Our plan at the beginning was to take another of our campus houses and make it into a temporary residence. But as the days passed this program seemed less and less feasible. The safety of the children had been guaranteed by the elaborate fire and smoke alarm system we had installed. It would be several weeks before such a plant could be added to an existing house; we did not want to go without it.

Then Ellen Lawson admitted that she really wanted to quit. The responsibility of these children was too great for her, she said. Even with all the help (she was very generous), the problems seemed too heavy for her to bear again. She had not realized, she said, just how tired she was. Now that the house was burned, she really did not feel able to start all over again.

So the complications continued. After a week— two weeks—we had to begin moving the children. After a month, I knew in my heart that we were not going to rebuild the residence. We had learned the hard way that mixing school and total care did not work for us. It demanded more human and financial resources than we could spare for the purpose.

Oh, we debated and considered, Dick Switzer and my board members and I. We kept delaying the issue, and we kept talking in "blue sky" terms about what ought to be done for these children. But all the while, Jack Taylor's warning that we were in over our heads was ringing very loudly in our ears. The insurance company was not pleased with the implication that one of the children had burned down the residence. The fire department was not pleased either— although nobody went so far as to term us a menace to community safety. But when we went about our business and ran our school we did not have these complications. Nor were we totally equipped to deal properly with such agencies as the Universal Association on a total-care basis. It was all something new, something that threatened to become more and more involving, at the expense of our tried and admirable system of education for the handicapped.

As the year came to a close, we were definitely on a new course, and one by one the children of the residence began to slip away from us.

Odd, is it not. While they were at the residence,

before it burned, some of them could think only of the pleasantries of their previous life. Now that the residence was gone, it seemed more like home to them than it ever had been while it operated. Yet it was a success, because it did instill those memories, and those children would gladly have gone back to try again to live in a more or less family atmosphere.

For a while they kept asking, and I kept smiling and assuring all concerned that it would work out in time. But then the people who had so kindly taken in these orphans of the storm began to grow a little restless. They had volunteered temporary services; we could not abuse their good nature too long. So one by one the children drifted off.

Susan went to a foster residence in Staten Island. That meant she would have to leave the school, because there was no way that we could arrange transportation that far. And Paula went with her. They ended up going to public school on Staten Island, and from what I last heard they adjusted very well, although they did continue to talk a great deal about the residence and the fire, and offer hope that sometime the plan would be brought back into being.

As for the boys, Gary and Michael were moved to a professional foster home in the Bronx. Michael was soon enrolled in a New York City school. Gary continued to attend Human Resources School. The New York system is good, although we think ours is better. The environment is right for Gary to progress, here. Michael never did learn to read, but at least in his new atmosphere he was put into a class with others his age and in a similar situation. He responded so well that one day a few years later when Dick went to visit the school, he found that Michael was president of the student council.

Nancy's story was more satisfactory to me. While she was in the hospital she met Mr. and Mrs. Alfred Di Nunzio, who had a child in the school, too. And when Nancy was well, the Di Nunzios took her to live with them and continue in Human Resources School. She began advancing through the grades.

All these changes came in a matter of weeks or months. And all the while, I was still talking about the repair and rebuilding of the residence, although I knew we were not going to do so. And the reason was that I was too concerned to destroy the hopes of all who so much wanted the residence continued. I wanted it myself, but one of the responsibilities of management is to look at the hard facts—and they told us we had no business running a "home."

One of our basic problems was the relationship with the welfare agency, and the strange, antiquated state regulations about foster homes. For example, a foster home has to deal with one agency; it can take a dozen children from the same agency if that is desirable, but they all have to be from the same agency. That might facilitate somebody's bookkeeping, but it creates a static situation that made a lot of trouble for Human Resources School, and so we felt we could not succeed, and must extricate ourselves from the foster-home field.

The real problem was to do so with as little interference as necessary in the lives and happiness of these children.

14

Adjustment

From being an occasional guest in the Kaley home to being a resident—even a temporary one—was a tremendous change for Darren. Now, suddenly he had a real family for the first time, built-in "grandparents," "parents" and two "sisters."

First of all, Darren had to have a room. Stefanie had been using a small room on the lower level of the split level house, for that way she could study late at night and her comings and goings would not upset the family. Stefanie gave up this room, and it became Darren's own. Of course Stefanie expected to reclaim it,

and of course, everyone in the family expected Darren
to be back at the residence before Spring.

But Chanukah came, and Darren was there for
the celebration. The Kaleys were not especially religious, but they did have special meals and candles for
the holiday table—they observed the high holidays,
and Passover—and Darren began to examine the etch-
ings of the Wailing Wall and other art work around
the house that represented the old traditions.

He learned to wipe his feet before coming into
the house, and to stay out of the living room except on
"occasions." He learned where the cookies were kept,
and managed the television all by himself. And best of
all—after school, he went out into the neighborhood
like any other little boy, and sought the other kids to
see what they were doing.

The whole epicenter of Darren's life changed in
that one day that he came to the Kaleys. Before, life
had been totally school-oriented. The residence was
an arm of the school—it was "run" that way, and
always the children felt that their center of life was
across the street. But now this house represented
family, and a solid place on the block. School for Darren, just as for the other youngsters he met in Syosset,
was someplace you went for the processes grownups
called education.

This time, Darren made real friends. The first
day was Wednesday, and most of school was missed
that day in all the excitement of the fire. The second
day was Thursday, and Darren had one new experience. Before, he would get up in the morning and have
his breakfast at the residence, and then walk over to
school with Todd when it came time for class. Now,

it was all different. He got up on Thursday morning, and got himself dressed except for tying shoes. Stefanie came in to be sure he had brushed his teeth and washed his face and combed his hair, and she tied his shoes.

It was about eight-thirty. She took him into the kitchen and made toast and oatmeal and milk for Darren and Alisa and herself. Mr. and Mrs. Kaley and the Dorskys got up earlier, for Mr. Kaley left at 8:30 for the office, and the Dorskys could never sleep late after all those years of running a restaurant in the garment district.

The bus came at nine. It was the first bus Darren had ever ridden in—a yellow van with a side ramp that reached the ground. Alisa had a van to herself, as she was the only child who came from this area of Syosset school district. Darren made two. He helped Alisa walk up the ramp, and then he got up front and rode with the driver, feeling very important to be there.

They got to school a little before ten. Darren jumped out, under the canopy that protected the bus from the weather, and ran back to help Alisa carry her books. The doors opened automatically into the long, low building, and the children were inside, Darren heading toward kindergarten, and Alisa toward the lockers and her own homeroom.

School ended late in the afternoon, and then it was home again on the bus. That was new and exciting enough for one day. Darren was still a little tired from the day of the fire, so he had a glass of milk and was happy enough to sit and watch TV for the rest of the afternoon, until Stefanie came home. She brought a brand-new coloring book, and together they sat under the lamp in the den and decided how to color the adventures of Yogi Bear in the forest. Then it was time for dinner, and time for bed, and a new day was ready to begin.

On the fourth day came another big change. It was Saturday, a cold Saturday in December, but bright and sunny nonetheless. That was the day Stefanie took Darren to the park again, and they met two small boys. Stefanie was wise enough to let Darren find his own way forward, while she hung back.

"What's your name?" asked Darren, jumping to the offensive.

"Scott," said the other. "This is my brother Chris."

"You're brown like me," said Darren.

"No we're not. We're Ceylonese, like Indian," said Scott.

"What's that?"

"You mean you don't know what India is? You don't know anything."

"Do too. Wanna fight?"

Seeing this turn of events from some ten feet back, Stefanie quickly intervened, and told Darren where India and Ceylon were and what they were. And with her interest and respect, Darren realized it was something different and important, and he lost his belligerency right there. In a minute the three boys were running through the park playing tag, and Stefanie was strolling along, keeping a benevolent eye on them.

This *was* a change. For these boys were not ephemeral—they lived around the corner from the Kaleys. They were Ceylonese, but they lived just like anybody, except that Mrs. Swaris liked to wear saris on special occasions, instead of ordinary ladies' dresses. And that was again something that had to be explained to Darren, and turned out to be a matter of much importance at kindergarten when he took in a picture of a sari for show-and-tell. And there were other strange adventures with the Swarises, such as dinner one evening on a special occasion. Lunch at the Swarises' was like lunch any place—soup and sandwiches, milk and cookies. But one night Darren came to dinner, and sampled dahl and curry, and rice cooked in the Ceylonese style. He liked dahl but he did not like curry and he hated ghee, the clarified butter that sits on every Indian table.

The family—the Swarises—were just like anybody, like the Kaleys and the McPhersons down the block whose son Jimmy was in first grade and therefore miles away from Darren and the little boys. But of course if it was a question of a game of ball, where bodies were needed, then the little kids were tolerated.

The interesting thing—Stefanie saw it from the very beginning—was the open interest with which these children first examined Darren, and then how they completely disregarded his appearance. He could give them a show with his plastic eye, and sometimes he took it out, but Stefanie explained that it was both unsanitary and showoff to be playing with his eye. He listened gravely, and after that first occasion when she chided him, he did not take out his eye in public again unless it came out under stress, which sometimes happened because the socket was too large.

These little problems began to endear Darren to the Kaley family. By Christmas time he was ensconced, I would say. Mrs. Kaley took him into New York to go shopping at Bloomingdale's.

What an experience!

The ride on the railroad from Syosset station into New York—seeing all those houses and all those people who crowded into the train on their way in to do their shopping. Sitting in a big seat with Mrs. Kaley, and remembering to keep his shoes off the seat and his coat unbuttoned so he would not catch cold when they went outside. Going into the tunnel underground that led to Pennsylvania station. Trying to get a drink of water all by himself at the end of the car. All those trains and all that track. And then the bumping and screeching as the car came to a halt in the long train, and they were at the station.

Grasping Mrs. Kaley's hand tightly so as not to get lost, taking the escalator up to the station floor and then another escalator out onto the street, and then the buses, to get to Bloomingdales.

Fifth Avenue with its Christmas decorations and busy crowds. All those yellow taxis. People jostling and rushing everywhere. And then Bloomingdale's. What a store! Dozens of counters, all glass and goodies inside. Bathroom smells, and pretty bottles. The toy department with its trains and bicycles and stuffed animals. In fact, the toy department will not soon be forgotten in the Kaley family, for that was where another little bit of history was made.

Darren was back in the forest of electric trains, looking them over with the practiced eye of an incipient expert, when up came another little boy whose mother was occupied with one of the clerks. The other was a small white boy, about Darren's size, dressed in a navy blue coat, blue cap, and black shoes that had "city" written all over them. The little boy came up to Darren and stared at him—Darren in his parka, already-scuffed shoes, and his blue corduroys. The boy first stared at Darren's clothes, and then he stared at the one eye and the twisted mouth.

Darren looked at him for a minute.

"Sit down," he said. "What are you staring at?"

"I was looking at your face. It looks funny."

"That's right," said Darren calmly, palming his eye. "There, see. I've got a false eye. Some people have false teeth too. Do you want to be friends? Or do you want to fight?"

"Be friends," said blue suit. "Lemme see the eye."

And so the little boy from upper Fifth Avenue was the first kid on his block to hold a nice big brown plastic eye in his own hand before Mother Kaley could hurry up and tell Darren to put the eye back where it belonged.

After that there was a good deal of train-looking and admiring of tin soldiers and traction motor cars and airplanes that could really fly. When the lady turned around to find the young man in the blue suit, he caught her eye, just as she was signing the last of the purchase receipts. The young man hastened over, one arm through Darren's to see his mother.

"Mother," said he. "This is Darren. He is my very best friend."

15
Every Day

Every day Darren woke up smiling, for every day brought a new adventure at the Kaley house. Now he celebrated both Chanukah and Christmas, for the Kaleys knew well that he would be brought up eventually in a Protestant society, not Jewish, and they must prepare him in the little time that they would have him. For Christmas that year there was a drum, and roller skates which could be used on the smooth blacktop surface outside, even better in the skating area of the park. There were puzzles, games and clothes. There was talk about a bicycle.

"But we're not millionaires," said Lou Kaley. "You know you don't buy a bicycle for $25 any more as it was when I was a kid. Now if he was going to stay with us. . . ."

But that was never in prospect. It had been made quite plain from the outset that we were asking the Kaleys only to do us a king-sized favor for a few days or at the most a few weeks. No, Darren was coming back to the residence just as soon as Dr. Viscardi and the others got things straightened out.

You live a little lie and it gets to you. It always happens.

Not that we started out by lying to the Kaleys. It was our intention, Dick's and mine, to reestablish the residence. There were times when I questioned the wisdom of such action. Others had to be consulted, the board was not nearly so enthusiastic this second time around, and as January came blowing snowily in, I knew in my heart that no matter how much I talked big, the chances of the residence being used again were growing slimmer every day. But it was the depth of winter, a holding time for all of us. When we saw Stefanie at the school we talked vaguely of spring and the plans for the future. And then when the residence had to be completely redone, in order to salvage the building, we talked bravely of late spring and all the changes.

The children talked as much as we. For a little time all six of the survivors of the residence were in school, and they spoke ever more wistfully it seemed to me and the teachers, of the days when they had played so happily in the house and all the fun they had had. That it wasn't necessarily so did not mar the dream, and we said nothing, but went about our various ways. One by one the girls and boys had to be told that the temporary arrangements must be abandoned, and that they would be going to other schools.

"But what about the residence?" they would ask.

"Give us a little time," we would say. "Give a little time—maybe a year or a decade or a hundred years" is what we were beginning to mean. For the cost picture became clear, the damage picture became clear, the conditions under which we would have to operate became clear, and by February, the dream of the residence existed almost entirely in the children's minds.

By this time I was shamefaced, and I suggested to Dick that he have a long talk with the Kaleys and see if they did not wish to move Darren to another family. "Just for a while," of course. But we felt the imposition was too great, for them to wait until the residence was rebuilt.

"We don't think that way," said Mr. Kaley. "This poor little child has been pushed around enough already. He's four and a half years old and he's lived in four different places. That ought to be enough for a while. No. We'll keep him until you're ready."

And of course we were not then ready to dash everyone's hopes by declaring that the residence would not be rebuilt for that purpose at all. Instead— the pressure was already on—it was going to be used as a dormitory for college interns. This was the kind of program that must appeal to a board: it gave us credentials with universities, it gave a training ground, and it provided additional help for the school when the school needed trained helpers. It would bring a new dimension to the undergraduates who would come on our campus.

So we delayed in telling the truth, and thus we lived a little lie. Luckily, time made it a white lie; it might have become another color under another set of circumstances.

But for Darren this was the finest life he had ever known. He had real playmates, kids down the block. Sure, they went to a different school, but so did some of the Catholic kids in the area. He was just another boy on the block, and after that first long look, nobody said a word about the ear and the eye and the diminishing harelip.

Some adjustment had to be made. Darren didn't have as much time to play outside as his peers on the block, because he had a double session at school. Mrs. Kaley was working part time, and Mr. Kaley spent his days working in Suffolk County. Stefanie had her car, and her own school responsibilities. So to go to school, Darren had to squeeze in on Alisa's run, which meant he had to stay all during the school day. That meant he went into the nursery school with the little ones in the morning and then into kindergarten with the older children at lunch time. Of course he had his mat and he took several rests, and Judy took a special interest and kept an eye on him. The fact that he was ambulatory made it a lot easier. The children in wheelchairs go through a tremendous physical strain every day in the process of going to school. Not so with Darren. He recognized it, and promptly appointed himself assistant teacher of both classes. He would run the teachers' errands and help put away coats and sort out lunches and sharpen pencils. He was a real help. And to think that less than a year earlier a shy little backward boy had been delivered to the residence from a home somewhere in the Bronx borough of New York City. Any relationship between that poor waif and this bright young boy was weighted for the future, not dimmed by the past.

Darren was all over the school. I could scarcely take a visitor through without seeing him. I could go for days without spotting some of the others, for they seemed to meld into the rooms and the furniture; but not Darren.

One day I was riding my little cart down the hall, when out of the kindergarten stepped Mrs. Steinberg.

"Just a minute, Hank," she said. "Darren wants to talk to you."

I looked inside. There he was, of all things, sitting *under* a desk. "He's hiding, to sneak up on you."

Just then, out from under his desk rushed Darren, and in his hand he carried a bow tie, of the tie-it-yourself-kind that I invariably wear to the office.

"Look what I got," he said. "Tie it for me."

So I stood in front of him and tied the tie. Only I didn't. I mean, it didn't. For years I have been tying neckties by feel and habit, and when I look at myself in the mirror it is all very natural. But this was all backwards, and I could not tie the tie until I got around behind Darren and pretended I was tying it on myself. Then it all came back to me and it worked.

It *was* a little odd. Darren was wearing a T-shirt, and the bow tie stuck up about two inches above the round collar on his neck. But he wore it that way, all the rest of the day, proud that he had a necktie of his own.

That evening, when Darren and Alisa had arrived at home from school, and Stefanie came home from Hofstra University, he was still wearing the tie. He and Stefanie wrestled for a while in the TV room, and then she read to him, and then it was time for dinner. He was still wearing the tie. And then came bedtime, and Darren got into his pyjamas and kissed everyone goodnight and went off to his bed in the little room downstairs. Later that evening Stefanie called in to check on him as she usually did before she went to bed. He was still wearing the tie.

The necktie was one of Lou Kaley's. Whatever happened to it no one can now remember, for once the excitement was over, Darren was much more comfortable in the clothes of a little suburban Long Island boy. But here came a little rub—for while the Kaleys were moderately well-off and lived by good middle-class American standards, the acceptance of a new person in the household brought new expenses, some of it anticipated, some not. We had never considered this aspect of the problem. Except for Abilities, Inc., our workshop which supports itself out of earnings, our activities are funded by donations and grants, and by various state, federal, and local programs in which we participate. A family does not have the same elasticity of budget that an organization can have. And soon the laxities of the welfare agencies began to cause some pain to the Kaleys.

We were all looking forward to the day when Darren would be housed elsewhere—the Kaleys thinking of the residence, and I knowing that he would have to go into a permanent foster home of some kind. So while Darren dearly wanted a bicycle, even with training wheels, or would have settled for a tricycle, the Kaleys did not feel it proper to engage in that kind of expense for so short a time. They were thinking in terms of weeks that winter.

Yet the weeks wore on and as spring came, so did the demand for changes in wardrobe. The Kaleys had outfitted Darren at their own expense. That was wrong from the policy point of view—they should be reimbursed. Darren was a ward of the public authorities. The public paid, or was supposed to pay, all his legitimate expenses. We at the school had never considered that any of our helpful parents would be saddled with extra expense in addition to all else they took on when they accepted a child for a time.

But the weeks went by, and the Kaleys had no reimbursement of any kind for anything regarding Darren. Indeed, the authorities did not seem too concerned about what had happened to him. They did not come to the school, even after we reported on the fire. They did not come to visit the family for a few months, to see how Darren was coming along.

Spring's coming precipitated the problem early in April. One afternoon Stefanie took Darren out into the garden to see the blooming daffodils and tulips, and to have a little lesson on plant culture and color. They looked at one flower and then another. They saw a stamen and a pistil, and Stefanie explained how one produced the pollen and the other the seed. And while they were out in the late afternoon sun, it turned a little chilly.

"That's all right, I'll get my coat," said Darren. And he rushed in and appeared a moment later in his big parka.

Then, two days later on Saturday, the Swaris boys came over with mitts and ball and bat to get Darren to play baseball in the park. He picked up his winter parka.

"Come on, that's too big," said one of the boys. "You can't play ball in that thing."

"But it's all I've got."

"Okay, then come on."

So they went out, and when Stefanie walked over to the park an hour later she saw Darren in his shirt sleeves in the nippy spring midmorning, playing baseball in the field. She felt like shouting at him to put on his coat, but she remembered what the boys had said, and was quiet. She waved, watched, and turned around to go home.

Her father was puttering in the basement, contemplating the dragging of hoses and the wheelbarrow and garden tools upstairs to the garage for the spring and summer months.

"Dad," she said. "Darren needs a jacket."

"I suppose he does," said Lou Kaley absently. "Then let's get him one."

"Are they awfully expensive?"

"These days they're not cheap."

"We really shouldn't have to pay."

"That's true. But let's get the jacket first."

That afternoon, Stefanie took Darren to the nearby shopping center and found a warm-up jacket with the symbol of the New York Mets. Just what a baseball player needed on these spring mornings.

Then, on Monday, from the office, Mr. Kaley made a few calls to the Universal Association offices. He was shunted from one place to another, even though we had given him our most up-to-date information about the telephone numbers and people who were "authority" in this case.

Next day, Lou Kaley tried again. And the next day once again, but he was getting nowhere by telephone. If he waited until the weekend, he would find no one in the welfare office. He did wait, and he called again, and he got precisely nowhere, except to learn that the man in charge of the division in which Darren's case was filed, was Mr. Grey, whose office was in the middle of the welfare building in Manhattan. Lou Kaley was finally given an appointment to see Mr. Grey.

Taking half a day off from his work, with apologies to those who worked under him, Lou Kaley went into Manhattan, to the office building where the Association was housed.

A hard walnut bench on a parqueted vinyl asbestos floor was against an institutional green wall decorated with a sign "No smoking." He sat down and waited. The anteroom was empty. The little glass window was untended. He must be too early. He waited half an hour. A passing friendly, matronly-looking woman asked him if she could help.

"No one ever mans that window any more," she smiled. "Cutbacks, you know."

Mr. Kaley stated his business to the friendly woman.

"I'll get someone to help you," she said, reassuringly, and went on inside.

Lou Kaley waited.

Half an hour went by, and no one came out. He gathered courage and opened the door. Inside, people were moving about, typewriters were clacking. He stopped at a desk and spoke to a Puerto Rican girl.

"I need to see Mr. Grey."

"Have you an appointment?"

"Yes, and I have been trying to reach him for a week. I can't get him to return a call."

"Just a minute. I'll see."

She went back into a glassed-in partitioned office, and spoke to a large, graying man for a moment. He looked up, saw Kaley, and immediately began shuffling papers.

The girl came back.

"I'm sorry. Mr. Grey isn't here today."

"Then I'll see somebody else. I want to talk about a case—Darren Dillard, a little crippled boy."

"I'm sorry. There's no one else."

Lou Kaley was now losing his patience.

"Look," he said. "I am going back out into the hall to wait. I shall wait until lunchtime. If nobody sees me by lunchtime I shall get on the subway and go down to City Hall and see the Mayor."

The girl took one look at his intense face, and listened to the quiet ferocity of his tone.

"Yes sir." she said. "I will see what I can do."

And she did, because in five minutes, a young man came out into the green hall where Mr. Kaley was sitting on his walnut bench counting the parqueted, black and white vinyl asbestos squares.

"Mr. Kaley?" he said. "Come right in. I understand you want to see us about one of our cases."

And within three-quarters of an hour, although the case worker had just been transferred and there was no one in the office who could even remember little Darren Dillard, the files were found, Mr. Kaley made his claim, and walked out of the office with a check that represented every penny he had spent, plus a monthly allowance for the care and upkeep of Darren. From that day on there were no further financial troubles with welfare.

16

The Decision

The Kaley family had never really expected to keep Darren Dillard for very long. Two children of their own were really quite a handful, when you considered everything. Stefanie's college education was going to be eight years long. She intended to become a psychologist, and that meant a Ph. D. And although Stefanie received a partial scholarship and aid as an undergraduate, still the expense was high.

Then there was the question of Alisa. Her expenses were very high, including medication and special equipment, and sometimes care. Alisa's dysautonomia had been diagnosed when she was three, and she was now sixteen. Although she made fine progress in our school, because of the environment and the teaching, she was still behind her normal age group because of the Brooklyn years. And she did demand a good deal of attention, although each month she was learning to do more for herself at school and at home.

The Kaleys did not complain. Theirs was a happy and loving family, made more tender and affectionate by the very trials they had faced. Lou Kaley worked hard for his company, and for the National Foundation for Dysautonomia, of which he was an officer.

They had certainly faced the difficulties. From the age of thirteen, Alisa had worn a steel brace from neck to waist, to correct a curvature of the spine. Now, she was much better off although she would still have to wear the brace for another several years. She could walk even without the brace, but to walk an entire city block demanded tremendous effort and concentration. And in the processes of dysautonomia, she had lost the sight of her left eye.

The coming of Darren meant that the whole family had to push over for "one more" and the process was hardest of all on Alisa. Before Darren's advent, Alisa was the center of family attention. Grandparents, parents and Stefanie all did their very best to make Alisa's lot a little easier. As was so often the case with our handicapped children, they tended to spoil her, to do things for her that she should have been capable of doing herself. But why not? They, in their robust health, felt a little guilty that one they loved should be deprived, and how better could one make it up to her than by little loving services?

Before Darren came to live with them, Alisa seemed to be getting on much, much better than before. I remember that when she first came to the school she was a problem. Like many dysautonomia children, she had temper tantrums. One day I was in Judy's office talking over some administrative matter when Alisa's teacher brought her in. Alisa's lower face was covered with blood.

"What happened?" I asked.

Judy spoke, directly to Alisa.

"You've been biting your lips again, haven't you?"

Whereupon she looked at the cuts, touched them up with hydrogen peroxide, and sent her back to class.

I looked at Judy. She seemed very casual about it all.

"Not too much sympathy, Hank," she said. "You cannot encourage temper tantrums around here. That's why I use hydrogen peroxide. It tastes terrible. And if she doesn't get sympathy and gets nothing but a bad taste, you'd be surprised at how quickly that lipbiting stops."

And of course Judy was right. Given real sympathy for her illness, and real encouragement for her willingness to catch up to the outside world, we saw Alisa prosper at our school in the late 1960s and early 1970s. By the time Darren came to us, Alisa was very nearly caught up with her age group and there was every indication that she would do just fine. She had made friends in school, and some on the block in Syosset—at least enough there that sometimes she talked wistfully of going out to regular Syosset school, and parents and teachers had to persuade her that until she was ready, she was better off with our special facilities. That's where our swimming pool helps a lot.

Stefanie was a real help. As soon as the family found out what ailed Alisa, Stefanie began treating her with grave tenderness and love. She even spoiled her little sister. And then, when Stefanie came to her graduate college years, and opted to become a psychologist, she found that right at home she had a part of her course. Her approach became a combination of clinical and sisterly love; no longer did she spoil sister Alisa so outrageously, but she demanded from client Alisa a good deal more self-management. And it worked. Alisa complained, then learned that she could do things for herself and liked the results, and the relationship just kept growing. Before, she stood off and bit her lips. Now she came to Stefanie and asked her to help solve problems. What about Syosset school? And when Stefanie agreed with parents and teachers that in a little while they would all be better able to discuss the change, Alisa accepted Stefanie's advice and was again content.

That's how it was in December, 1972, when Darren first came to stay with the Kaley family.

At the end of the first month, Alisa began to grow a little restless. Stefanie had seen her sister biting her lip again at the table, when a last bit of cheese cake had been given to Darren instead of to Alisa. Always before the delicacies were Alisa's little pleasure, the extras of everything. Now there was competition.

She had complained to Stefanie, but Stefanie had only laughed.

"Come on, Lisa," she had said. "He's just a little

boy. And he's only going to be here for a little while. Don't get mad."

And Alisa had listened and smiled, and had forgotten all about the cheese cake.

But in February Darren was still getting the best of everything. On the night that Mrs. Kaley and Stefanie had gone out to buy Darren some new clothes, Alisa complained.

"How come he gets everything?"

"You got a new dress and new shoes. What are you worrying about?"

"How come he gets a jacket and all this stuff?"

"He needs it. That's why. You're not paying for it, so stop worrying."

"Darren gets everything around here."

"That's not nice, 'Lisa. You'll hurt his feelings."

"I don't care."

That was not true, and Stefanie knew it. For except at the times when Darren annoyed her by his presence and threat to her position, Alisa liked him. He was a sweet little boy. He rushed to get Alisa's pills for her in the evenings, and brought her glasses of water in bed so she would not have to get up, and he helped get her books ready for school in the morning —all those things that are hard for a handicapped person, things that involve picking up and moving about. So Alisa really liked the little brown boy, too.

But Stefanie was worried more about something else as April rolled in. She felt that her mother was under too great a strain. Mrs. Kaley had helped the family income by part-time bookkeeping for the past three years. So that she could do that, the Dorskys pitched in with the housework. Taking care of Alisa always took a good deal of effort on the part of several members of the family. Her washing was always meticulously done, and her clothes were always clean and neat. That did not happen by accident; the simple problem of hanging up and retrieving was an effort that someone had to make.

In this spring of 1972, the problem of an extra person to care for became difficult for Mrs. Kaley, and in another way as well. The Kaleys had scarcely ever gone anywhere by themselves, even overnight. For years they had spent summers in the Catskills—family vacations—taking mountain cottages where the girls could enjoy the fresh sweet smells of the countryside and the whole family could leave, for a while, the strident grating of city life. But that was not the same as "getting away from the kids," and the Kaleys had never done that.

In the spring of 1972, they decided to try. One day Mr. Kaley came home from work with a handful of brightly colored folders.

"What have you got there, Lou?" asked Mrs. Kaley.

"How'd you like to go to London. . . . the Tower . . . big Ben. . . . Beefeaters. . . . . cathedrals. . . . . changing the guard. . . . ?"

Mrs. Kaley seized them and sat down at the table in the kitchen.

"You don't mean it." Already she was leafing like a diner inside a menu.

"I do mean it."

"Sure." Then came second thoughts. "But what about the children. Alisa. . . . Darren?"

"Darren may not be with us that long. He's supposed to go on back any time now. And your mother and father and Steffie certainly should be able to take care of Alisa for a week."

"I don't know. . . . . . . I don't know. . . . . ."

But in the end, Mrs. Kaley's reluctance was overcome and she was persuaded.

Still, Stefanie could tell that her mother was worried at the prospect of leaving the household unattended for even a week.

Stefanie worried. Stefanie fretted. Stefanie thought.

One day, about two weeks before the flight was scheduled, Stefanie came to her mother in the evening and sat down at the kitchen table.

"Mom, when you're gone, I want to have Alisa take some responsibility for Darren."

"Alisa? What can she do?"

"She can check his room and see that he picks up his clothes. She can be sure the den is cleaned up before she goes to bed at night and all those toys are put away. She doesn't have to clean up after him. She just has to make sure he does his jobs."

So Mother Kaley agreed, although she was not at all sure how it would work out, and then the parents went away to enjoy themselves for their week of freedom from care.

Stefanie's psychology instructors had taught her well. For at the end of the week, when the Kaleys returned, the household was not only serene, it beamed with good will and love. Alisa was learning the beauties of being able to take care of someone other than herself.

Coming as it did, that revelation brought the Kaleys to thinking hard again about the future of the little black boy that fate had cast into their house.

And all this time we were going through the throes at the school and at Human Resources Center in general. We kept saying that it would be a foolish thing to rebuild the residence. And we were already losing the children who had been burned out; their temporary "homes" were disappearing one by one, and, as they had to be found new residences, the youngsters were being moved, by the Universal Association, out of our region and away from our school.

One day it came to a head. We just could not get along well enough with the agency. We knew that if we were to have children living on our grounds, we would have to have control of their accomodations, so we could bring them up so that they could realize the real goals of their lives. And it all boiled down to that. To do so, we would have to embark on a whole new struggle through the bureaucratic machinery in order to have agency status and take responsibility for children. If we did that, the demands on us would be so great to take on new children, that we might very well endanger all that we were trying to do in the educational field.

The nagging had to come to an end, and it did in a board meeting. Next day, I called the Kaleys and told them what had been decided, and that we must find a home for Darren and prepare to move him.

It was one of the saddest moments of my life, and I could tell by Lou Kaley's voice that he was nearly as shaken as I was. But there were the facts. What else could we do?

17
The Family

On the day that I telephoned the Kaleys, it was just as well that I could not be a little mouse and overhear the conversations that occurred at the family dinner table. Not that anything was said about me, or anything unkind about the school. In fact, very little was said about anything. The room was unusually silent, and the two younger children could not understand why the adults were suddenly so glum. Stefanie had been taken into her parents' confidence, and she was unhappiest of all, for she felt that if she had not become involved with Darren, he would be much better off. His whole future would have been decided months ago. He would be with a permanent foster home by now, and he would have the love and settling-in that he needed.

For, of course, Darren knew all the time that he was scheduled to go back to the residence. For that reason he had held back a little with Scott and Chris Swaris and his other friends. He could not think ahead more than a week at a time.

"Am I going back to the residence next week?" he would ask Stefanie every Saturday.

And every Saturday Stefanie would shake her head.

"No, not this week, Darren," she would say. "Maybe next week. We'll see."

But now, Darren knew that something was being decided and, even as the family talked over the next step, he stopped asking when he was going back to the residence. Mr. Kaley believed it was because he was becoming so well adapted here in Syosset. Stefanie knew—the real reason was the sorrowful knowledge that his fate was hanging in the balance, and that what was likely to happen to him was still unknown. It was enough to make her cry. And it became worse when the Kaleys suggested, and I concurred, that Stefanie, with all her studies, her experience, her knowledge, and with her love for little Darren—that she should be the one to find the family that would take him. We did not know then that we were wrenching at Stefanie's heart.

Night after night she would lie awake, worrying about what she must do. "Who am I to be deciding what this boy will have for a life?" she asked herself.

"What right do I have to make such a decision?"

But Stefanie was true to her word. She had said she would search for a home for Darren, and she did. She and I agreed that we should keep Darren in the school zone if we could—and that meant finding him a nearby home on Long Island—for the local school district would then provide transportation, and that was a basic requirement of the school.

All this while Stefanie was keeping her own heart in mind as well. She made sure that the people she saw would be favorable to a little black boy. It was not whether they were black or white that mattered, but their kindliness of heart. And this was what she searched for, high and low. She was also interested in making sure that she could visit Darren again after he was "placed." But love and tenderness were the objects of the search.

By now Darren knew all. One day a social worker from the Association contacted the Kaleys and came out to inspect their house, and especially Darren's room.

Nodding and nodding and nodding to answer the barrage of questions, Mr. Kaley showed the lady the little room on the ground floor where Darren stayed.

"Of course the boy has the run of the whole house," he said.

"Good. But that doesn't matter," said the social worker. "Doesn't matter at all. We've got requirements. Just the room. That's a most important thing that we check."

So the lady got to Darren's room and got down on her hands and knees, and pulled a round metal tape out of her pocket and began to measure and figure.

When she was finished, she got up and put the paper and tape in her pocket and started out the door.

"Well," said Mr. Kaley.

"Well what?"

"Does it meet the requirements?"

"Yes, it does."

"That's fine."

"Goodbye." And the lady was off and into her car and away for her next tapemeasuring job.

That night at the dinner table Mr. Kaley told his story.

"It was odd," said Mr. Kaley.

"Why do you say that?" asked Alisa.

"Because I'm not going to be here very long," said Darren, mustering a wan smile.

Stefanie suddenly left the table, and put her napkin over her face and ran out of the room. Father Kaley and Grandfather Dorsky looked at one another. Mother Kaley half rose then sank back in her chair, shaking her head. Alisa bobbed her head toward her plate. And Darren ran away from the table and into Stefanie's room to comfort her.

Somehow, though, the little tension that was building was erased by this outburst. Darren now approached the subject very calmly.

"Do you think you can find a house as nice as this, Steffie?" he asked her. "Do you think I'll have any little kids like me to play with?"

"Would you like to be in a family with children your age?" Stefanie asked.

"That would be fun."

It was obvious by May that Darren had accepted the fact that he must leave the Kaleys. It made no difference to his attitude toward them, at least none that we could ascertain. Yet—what must have been going on in that little head, rejected by one family after another? Living on borrowed time in a place that he loved, and where he was receiving love and attention every day. He was just over five years old now. What a burden for so small a child!

The knowledge made Stefanie's own burden that much heavier. She tried very hard. She found one family after another, and either she rejected them or, when they discovered that Darren was black, or that he was physically disfigured in the way he was, they rejected him.

That was fine. She did not want anyone who would go into the foster-family affair for money, without regard for the little boy they were going to take into their home. There was more than enough of that in the world already.

May sped by. Toward the end of the month, Stefanie found a family for Darren. The Redfearns. Everything was right. It was a black family, living in Westbury, not too far from the Kaley house. The Redfearns were fine people. Mr. Redfearn worked for one of the county departments. They had one son who was in high school at Human Resources School, another teen-age boy, and two girls eight and three. Darren would fit right in. The family had no apparent prejudices nor any worries about a little boy who was going to need plenty of medical work in the months to come —and a great deal of love to make it all bearable.

All went well. Darren was taken to visit the Redfearns and although nothing was said, he knew. On the way home he spoke to Stefanie.

"Are the Redfearns Jewish?"

"Why no." The concept startled her.

"Then I can't go to Temple."

She laughed outright.

"No, you can't go to Temple. You'll be going to a Protestant church. That's what your mother was— Protestant."

"I know it's a religion. But what is it?"

Stefanie threw up her hands and then hugged him to her. "I'm not a genius, Darren. I can't remember all these complicated things."

"Well, you find out about Protestants. I like Temple."

For several days it seemed that the proper place had been found at last; then "authority" raised its head once more. In addition to their own four children, the Redfearns had little Vivian, a two-year-old girl who was also a foster child. She had come to them from one of the county agencies. Darren was a Protestant—his papers said so—but his affairs were controlled by the Universal Association for Children, that had taken him in originally.

Stefanie had been told that the law stated that a family could have as many as ten foster children if they wished to care for so many, but that they could deal with but one agency. So the Redfearn house was out for Darren, for now.

The news did not upset the Kaleys as much as it might have. Stefanie met a newscaster at one of Human Resources' Easter Seal Telethons. She spoke with him about this legal problem. He assured her that he himself would work it out if she thought the Redfearns would be good for Darren. She did.

The legal and bureaucratic processes began. They dragged on for weeks. In that time Darren went to the house several times. He already knew the children. Stanley, the second son, played baseball in the park with the gang although he was nearly thirteen years old, and disappeared to play with the bigger boys whenever they showed up. So this household was most promising of all.

Legally, we at the school were never responsible for Darren and the other children, but when the legal complications began to be unravelled that spring, I had a call from the welfare people telling me it looked as though this transfer was going to work out all right. I happened to see Stefanie in the hall at school that day and I told her. Instead of happiness I got sadness. I sensed right then and there that the matter would come to a head within a few hours. And it did.

Stefanie went home that afternoon and told her father and mother what I had said.

"That's nice," said Mrs. Kaley. "For Darren."

"Yes," said Mr. Kaley. "It will be wonderful—for Darren."

And then they were very quiet.

Just before dinner, Stefanie saw her mother and father in very serious conversation out in the garden. They spoke emphatically to one another for a few minutes. Then they came in smiling.

"Stef," said Father Kaley, "what would you think about it if we decided we wanted to keep Darren here?"

Stefanie erupted in a shriek of joy. She danced on the kitchen floor and she threw her arms around her father, and her mother. "Oh, Dad—Mom—I can't tell you how happy that will make us! Darren will be so pleased. And me. And I am sure Alisa too. Oh this is great!"

So that night there was a party at the Kaley house, with ice cream and cake, and with an air of joy that blew away the clouds that had been gathering as everyone worried about the day that Darren would leave.

Next day, Stefanie came in to give me the news, all smiles and laughter.

"You know what Mother said the reason was when they told me? She said it was because of all those dreadful operations that Darren was going to have to have, and how awful it would be for him to have to come out and not have anybody to take care of him who really loved him."

18

The Operation

Stefanie contacted the March of Dimes, and was referred to the North Shore Hospital. There, in the Child Development Center, the first of Darren's next operations was scheduled for July. They were to be very important to Darren's future. The doctors said so, Stefanie knew it, and the Kaleys agreed that if Darren's speech patterns could be improved twenty-five percent by the harelip operation, these operations would mean everything to him. The doctor indicated that the first surgical effort would be on his cheek, and so sophisticated were the techniques of modern times, that he could very nearly guarantee a successful effort. Darren's bone structure on the left side of his face had not been completely formed at birth. The doctor was going to insert an artificial cheek bone into his left side. The doctor would also be attempting to straighten out Darren's malformed left ear lobe. This was the only part of the ear with which he was born. The Kaleys would tell Darren just about what he could expect, with almost every prospect that it would come true. Doctors and families are not always so very lucky as that. The surgeons showed infinite kindness toward Darren and the Kaleys, using every possible means to ease the situation for them.

As for the second operation, it was part of a longer process. The doctors would undertake two procedures at the second session. They would improve his artifical eye socket and, at the same time, they would begin the process of building up cartilage so that he could have an ear. In addition, they would insert a rubber prosthesis in the form of an ear. It was quite a lot to manage, but the doctors knew as well as anyone, that a little boy could not spend all his time in hospitals, that Darren's general health was fine and he was growing fast, and that his recuperative powers were excellent.

So the dates were made six months apart.

The second operation took much more of the attention of the whole family than did the first operation. The doctors took Darren into surgery in the morning and they did the operation on the side of his head that began the creation of the ear he had never had.

It was painful, and when Darren came out of the

anesthetic he was whimpering. Roslyn Kaley sat with him, and would wet his lips with water when he so requested. Lou Kaley, Stefanie and the rest of the family also came as often as they could. Darren was there for a whole week; by the end of the third day he had captivated the nursing staff, and by the fifth day he was bouncing in and out of his bed so that the doctors said they discharged him early just to keep a little order on the pediatrics floor.

"Otherwise he might be running the hospital," said the chief resident to Mrs. Kaley as he patted Darren on the shoulder and escorted them to the elevator on the day of the discharge.

There was still a little pain, and Darren was still in bandages around the ear, but all was very well indeed.

It had been just before the first trip to the hospital that Aunt Mary and Uncle Louie came to call one day. They were Roslyn Kaley's aunt and uncle, really, old-line members of the Jewish community of Queens, and they had certain prejudices that had been intensified in recent years as black people had moved inexorably into the old Jewish section of the borough. They came for dinner, and all morning long Roz Kaley and Grandmother Dorsky were cooking, touching up the linens with the handiron, and vacuuming and dusting the house.

Noon came, and the Chernins arrived in their car, from Queens. Darren was over at the park playing ball. The adults sat around the living room for an hour, drinking wine and talking about the old days in Brooklyn. Then Aunt Mary spoke up.

"Where is this little boy?"

"You mean Darren."

"Yes the little black boy you've taken in." She rolled her eyes. "A pity that you should be so foolish. What do you need this for?" And, not stopping for an answer, she was off on the merits of the drapes, the rug, and how much better were the furnishings one could still buy in Queens.

Roslyn Kaley watched her husband very carefully for signs of impending storm. But he was laughing, and so she laughed too.

After the wine, Stefanie went to the park to find Darren, and she brought him back, all hot and sweaty from his baseball game.

"Baseball? Five years old? Precocious," announced Aunt Mary, and Stefanie brightened as she took Darren into the bathroom to clean up before dinner.

But as she emerged, she frowned.

". . . and I don't understand how you could be so foolish. So I work all day for Hadassah. Okay. Still, you don't take it home with you at night. But a little one with no eye and no ear—" she shrugged amply, "and black. . . ." She shrugged again.

Somehow they all got through the meal, and nothing was said in front of Darren that would embarass him. That part was all right. Aunt Mary and Uncle Louie got into their car amid a cloud of cigar smoke and left for Queens.

The whole family went into the house to clean up and relax.

"Boy, do grown-ups talk," said Darren.

"Boy, do they ever," grinned Steffie.

But that night after Darren was in bed, Roz and

Lou Kaley worried over the incipient problem. They had really not considered the neighbors. How were they going to react to the Kaleys' bringing a black boy into what was essentially a lily-white society? To be sure there were the Swarises, but they were Ceylonese, not black, and although the Kaleys had never given the matter much thought, neither did anyone recall seeing more than one or two black faces in the parks or on the streets around the house. There were many Jewish families in the neighborhood. Would they react as had Uncle Louie and Aunt Mary?

That kind of thinking can be destructive. Stefanie went to bed wondering about her own motivation. For she knew that she, and she alone, was responsible for the continued presence of Darren in the house. There had been the beginning, when Mrs. Kaley had been most unsure of the whole experiment, and Stefanie had risen to the occasion, had taken on the extra work load, had spent hours and hours wrestling and coloring and watching TV with Darren, so he would not be a burden on the family.

Why? What was her motive?

In her mind, possible motives raced along like sheep to a crossing. Did she have to prove her own liberalism to somebody? She did not think so. No, it was the winsome little face that had first attracted her, that one great alive brown eye that followed her across the room, the whole face lighting up, and the fleeting graceful gestures of head and neck that belied the ugliness of eye and mouth and ear. She had known from the beginning that this little boy could be saved and she had wanted to be a part of it.

Sternly she suppressed a desire to turn over and

cry and feel sorry for all of them. Nonsense. They had nothing to feel sorry about. They were lucky to be alive and healthy and in the land where they lived. In three days now, Darren would head for the hospital, and the real job of reconstruction would begin. Sorry? She should be glad, for she was a part of the preservation of a person. And how well she knew, for in this last year of school she had begun interning in psychology, and was getting a shuddering view of the underside of American society. Little Darren would never have to face what she was seeing every day—dreadful housing and poor people roaming the streets because they had nothing else to do. No, the Kaleys had nothing of which to be ashamed, and everything of which to be proud.

So thinking, Stefanie fell asleep, and when she wakened next morning all the doubts were gone, nor did they ever return.

And three days later Darren did go to the hospital. The operation on his cheek was an unqualified success. He came out of the anesthetic smiling, with Stefanie sitting by his side in the recovery room. He touched his face, where the bandages were taped on.

"Hurts," he said thickly.

She hugged him. "It will hurt for a few days. But think of how handsome you will be. Maybe just like daddy."

"And then I'll have a mustache like Uncle Louie. Only bigger." He put out his hands to shape a handlebar mustache.

"Of course you will. Any kind of mustache you want, Darren," she said, and a tear came down to splash on her hand as she thought of what a wonderful life it would be for the little boy when all the surgical procedures would be completed.

Darren grinned then, and took her hand tightly in his own little brown fist, and in a moment he was fast asleep.

19

Busy Summer

July was a busy month for the Kaleys and Darren Dillard. There were decisions to be made, and excursions to go on just as soon as Darren got the bandages off his face and could move about outside the house.

What a difference! Even with the crooked red scar of the operation still showing a little, Darren's cheek was almost filled out. Of course, every two years until Darren stopped growing, a new artificial cheek bone would have to be implanted. But what a difference it made even now. Darren became so vain that he looked in the mirror for minutes on end to examine the changes.

"You think they'll make that eye like the other?" he asked Stefanie. They stared in the bathroom mirror and he wiggled his right eyebrow like Groucho Marx.

"They sure will. And that ear too."

"Then I *will* look like your father." For it was family belief—and truth—that Lou Kaley was a very handsome man.

And Stefanie laughed, with no choke in the throat at all, as she looked at what would be.

The Kaleys went to the Universal Association for a visit, and filled out the forms that would make them the official foster parents of Darren. And there the officials brought up another point.

"Ahem. . . ." said Mr. Grey. "What do you intend to do about the boy's religious education?"

"He will go to church. We will see to that."

"It says here (and Mr. Grey consulted a form), that his mother was a member of the Baptist church. Is there a Baptist church nearby?"

Stefanie sensed that they were treading on very dangerous ground. "I can certainly find one," she said. "I will see that he is entered in Sunday school when the time comes."

"And er . . . church attendance?"

"I will guarantee that he will be taken to services at a Baptist church on a regular basis. All along he has been attending a Protestant religious instruction class at Human Resources School."

"That will be just fine," said a relieved Mr. Grey. "Very fine indeed."

When they got outside, Darren turned to Stefanie. "Does that mean I couldn't go to Temple when you go?"

"Do you want to?"

"Of course I do. That's where the family goes. And I'll go to the Baptist thing too. . . ."

So it was done.

And so were many other things.

Permanence. It meant a bicycle. A very small bicycle with training wheels, and the truth is that Darren was not big enough this summer to really manage it. But he had talked so much about a bicycle, and the Swaris boys had bicycles and so did all the other bigger boys on the block. Lou Kaley and Stefanie went to the bicycle store with Darren, and they found one that he could get up on and reach the pedals, even though they were just a little long.

"He'll grow into it," said the salesman. "Training wheels are just the thing."

So the bicycle was bought. A beautiful machine of blue and white, with racing tires and silvery spokes and curved handlebars and a bell. They took it home in the back of Mr. Kaley's car and put it on the front walk. Stefanie guarded and helped while Darren had his first ride on the new bike.

He fell off.

He fell off half a dozen times and skinned his elbow, and had to be taken inside the house to be patched up with merthiolate and a Bandaid. But not a whimper. When you fall off a bike, that is part of the learning process, nobody is supposed to cry about that.

But after an hour, Darren could ride in a wobbly sort of way, and as long as Stefanie was around to guide him and keep an eye out for walkers on the sidewalk, it went all right.

She saw that he was tiring. The tip of his tongue was out between his teeth and it was a strain to push the pedals.

"All right," said Stefanie. "Enough for today."

"How about tomorrow?" No complaint. He knew. But tomorrow was a whole new world.

"Afternoon. When I get back from school."

So tomorrow became today and another ride was accomplished. And the next day, and the next. Until after a week, when the Swarises came by with their bikes, Mother Kaley felt secure enough to give Darren permission to ride with them as long as they stayed on that quiet circle drive and did not cross the intersections.

Darren knew. Those were *rules*, to be obeyed. There were no incidents.

Somehow, on the day that Darren's residence with the Kaleys was affirmed by the agency, the word flashed across the neighborhood telegraph. Before, Darren had been tolerated in the games in the park. Now, suddenly the magic of belonging was his, and boys came by the house in the mornings to collect him to make a game. Sometimes Mother Kaley packed a lunch and he and the Swarises stayed in the park half the day and then came home dirty and tired, but happy.

It was not all cookies and cake, however. Darren had his ups and downs like the rest of them. The first *down* that came to the attention of the Kaleys occurred about two weeks after Darren was home from his cheek operation.

He came dragging in later in the afternoon, and found Stefanie studying in her room.

"I gotta wash my hair," he said. "Will you help me?"

Odd request. Doubly odd from a little boy who hated baths as much as most.

"Why do you have to wash your hair?"

He was in a hurry. "Some kid threw sand in it."

Stefanie stopped.

"Now wait a minute. Have you been fighting?"

Darren's head went down, and his lower lip came out. He looked carefully at the tips of his shoes.

Stefanie repeated the question. "Well?"

The head came up, mouth turned down. "A little bit."

"All right. Now we'll go into the bathroom and wash your hair and you'll tell me all about it."

So they did. Darren's hair, like that of many blacks, is thick, and sand does not come out easy. So it was wash and scrub and rinse and wash again, while the story came out among the suds.

Darren had headed for the park that day to find Scott and Chris and his other friends, and there they were. So they had played ball for a while, and tag, and then just lay back on the green grass under the trees. They watched the sun shine through the white fleece of the clouds and the birds circling over head—the kind of watching that is pleasant when you are tired from a long game, and it was not quite time to go home in the lengthening shadows.

"Then up came this strange kid—nobody ever saw him before—ow, you got soap in my eye—hey that hurts—and. . . ."

"And what?"

"Wait'll I get the soap out. . . . And he looked at

my eye and he said what's wrong with your eye, kid?"

"And what did you say?"

"Well he made me so mad I said it was none of his business."

"And the kid just kept bugging me. He kept saying what's wrong with your eye, kid? So finally I said I had an operation."

"And then what did he say?"

"He said 'I don't care if you did,' and that made me madder. So I said 'Well my mother cares.' And he said 'Who cares about your mother?' And that made me so mad I socked him and he socked me back and picked up a lot of sand and threw it at me. And he started chasing me and I ran all the way out of the park and came home."

"What happened to Scott and Chris? Didn't they help you?"

"Come on, Steffie! Kids don't do things like that. It was this kid and me. He was biggern me."

"Than I."

"Okay, I. Are you almost through?"

And she was. So she dried the little brown head with a towel, and took Darren into his room to change his wet shirt for a dry one. The incident was forgotten. For as Darren reported it, the next time he saw the other boy, they got so chummy that Darren took out his false eye for the other, to show him how it worked.

If the Kaleys had any worries about integration in the neighborhood, by midsummer they were totally forgotten. And as for the Kaleys, to put it in the vernacular, they were completely "hooked" by this small black boy with all his facial problems. That summer,

Dick Switzer told me one story about the Kaleys and Darren that indicates how it was.

Darren was a member of our summer school camp. But he would rather play in the park, and we could understand that because this was his first year of real freedom. It would be wonderful if all our children at the school could spend their summers with children who are not handicapped, but with most of them their ambulatory difficulties and physical problems make it impossible. Darren's situation was unique, and we welcomed the chance for him to be out instead of in our camp. Yet there were attractions here. He liked to come sometimes with Alisa when the bus picked her up to bring her to the school for the summer program. So he did. And there was another reason—he had become enamored of Dick Switzer's daughter. "I'm going to marry her when I grow up," he told Dick confidentially that summer. And when Dick questioned his daughter, she said solemnly that she was going to marry Darren.

The Switzers got quite a kick out of those declarations. They also developed a very soft spot in their hearts for Darren, and prompted by their daughter, one weekend they asked him to come out "real camping" with them. The Switzers are camping bugs; they have a camping trailer and take excursions around the woods and countryside on weekends in the summer whenever Dick can get away. So one August weekend, Darren was formally invited to go along.

What excitement! The Kaleys made sure Darren had a pocket knife—that occasioned a trip to the hardware store. They checked over his sneakers and his blue jeans and borrowed Lou Kaley's sleeping bag and sent along some cookies and candy bars and a dollar for Darren to spend if they got near a store. Darren and Mr. Kaley got into Mr. Kaley's car on the morning that Darren was to be delivered, and they went to the Switzers' house next to the school. Darren got out, and Mr. Kaley waved as they said good bye.

And then it was off on the camping trip, which, this day, was to a state park out near the end of Suffolk county. Darren went to the beach with the Switzers and they went clamming with a big clam rake, and dug the clams and ate them steamed over a campfire. Yes, they had a real campfire as well as cooking on a Coleman stove on a picnic table. They roasted hot dogs and they told stories and that night they had a marshmallow roast, too. Darren really liked it—that is until it came time to go to bed, and for the first time that day he thought about "home" and the Kaleys and his own bed.

And during the night, Dick Switzer heard a sound like a puppy whimpering. He got up and found that Darren was crying softly in his sleeping bag.

"What's wrong?" he said, flashing the big flashlight.

"I was just thinking about home. I miss my mother and Steffie, and Lisa, and all the rest."

So Dick Switzer patted Darren on the shoulder and told him there would only be one more night and that, yes, everybody got homesick the first time, and that everything was going to be just fine and tomorrow they might see some deer.

"And a bear?"

"Well probably not a bear—but *maybe* a bear. A small one."

So sadness changed to joyful speculation about bears and Darren stopped sniffling and his thoughts marched off to sleep like a good boy's.

They did not see any bears the next day, since the bear population of Long Island is distinctly limited, but they were busy campers doing any number of things including fishing, and Darren quite forgot about his homesickness of the night before. But when they returned to Albertson on Sunday evening, and the Kaleys were called to say that they were home and Darren could be collected, the whole Kaley family came by in Mr. Kaley's car, including Alisa, and Stefanie jumped out and embraced Darren as he came around and kissed every one of them hello.

"That's how much love there is in that home," said Dick in wonderment as he told me the tale.

For after only these few months, Darren was totally ensconced as a member of the Kaley family, a late child who came to this middle-aged couple sixteen years after the birth of their second daughter.

So August was upon us—a worrisome August for Stefanie, for it meant more testing of the relationship. She had planned a trip to Europe with some friends for two weeks for that August of 1973—all this done early in the spring before Darren's relationship with the Kaleys was firmed up. Now, to go meant that she would be leaving Darren and her parents. Was it too much to ask of Mother Kaley and her father that they take this responsibility? For one of the promises that Stefanie had made when she brought Darren into the house for those first few nights, was that the boy would be no trouble, for she would take total responsibility for his care and behavior.

She mentioned it to her mother.

"Now, Steffie," said her mother, a little crossly, "that is being a silly, selfish girl. For Darren is just as much a part of our side of the family as he is of yours. We love him. We want to take care of him too."

And Stefanie saw then that she had been looking at the relationship only through her own eyes, not through the eyes of her father, and mother, and grandparents, and of Alisa, all of whom saw it differently. It was Darren's bright little soul that showed through in its own way and attracted him to all of them, all with their different needs and different reactions.

So Stefanie was content, and she went off to ooh and aah at cathedrals and rivers and great old buildings without a care in the world. They all missed her, but it was so busy a time that they probably did not miss her as much as she might have thought they did.

20

The Judge's Decision

Stefanie came home so brown from her trip that Darren looked at her in awe.

"Mommy is white and Grandma is white, but you're just like me, Steffie," he said, grinning.

And Stefanie broke down. Obviously there was no tension built up in the house, as she was afraid there might be. The thought had dogged her on the flight home, but as the family met her at Kennedy Airport and she saw how Darren and her mother held hands as they walked her from the gate, she knew all was well. There were no questions to be asked.

It was a new life for Stefanie. The European trip had been her present for graduation from Hofstra University; now she was entering another furious four years, going into a Ph.D program of accelerated work in psychology at Hofstra. And now that she was "grown up" there were new concerns.

Darren had been talking to his peers in the park that summer. Stefanie's name had come up, and he had announced proudly that she was in Europe.

"What's she doing there?" asked Scott Swaris.

"She got it for graduation."

"Graduation, huh. Then she's gonna get married. That's what they do."

"Gee," said Darren, who had never really considered that possibility.

This fall, as school started once again and young men appeared at the house in the evenings to "take Steffie out," Darren began regarding them with a jaundiced eye. It was something of a shock for a college student to come to pick up his date and find himself examined carefully by a small black boy with a false eye and only part of an ear. But that did not stop Darren from giving them sharp scrutiny.

One day after a date of the night before, Darren spoke up as he and Stefanie were having breakfast.

"You gonna get married?"

She looked at him sharply. "I suppose so some day. Why?"

"Scott says you're gonna get married. That's what girls do."

She laughed. "Well, that's true more or less. Yes, I will get married when I find the right young man."

"How about that one last night?"

She laughed again. "I don't think so. Say, what's this third degree all about?"

"He didn't like me. I could tell. And I didn't like him either."

Stefanie examined Darren closely. How shrewd he was. For as they were driving to the movies, the young man in question had asked her how in the world the family ever got mixed up with a "kid like him." And of course that had set the tone for what turned out to be a thoroughly miserable evening.

She laughed ruefully. "Maybe I had better let you screen my dates. I didn't like him either."

"What's screen?"

Stefanie picked up her coffee cup. "Forget it, Darren. That was just a big people's joke. I'll be around for a long time yet."

"That's good. Because when you get married I want to get married too. I'll go with you."

Yet after school had been on for a month, Stefanie could see a gradual change in the family. Darren was no longer so dependent on her. When the question of her dates and marriage came up, he did not seem overly interested.

"Sure," he said one night. "You're going to get married and leave home. Lisa and I will be around here a lot longer than you."

So he was adjusting. And the reason of course was the firm entrenchment of the little black boy in the hearts of the white Jewish parents and grandparents. He *knew* he was wanted; no one had to say a thing to him. He knew he was happy. And when he and Alisa quarreled, over the use of their favorite chair in the den, why, it was a new kind of bickering—the "I got here first" kind—and Alisa no longer regarded Darren as a stranger who was threatening her position, but as a sibling with whom one was expected to have a certain amount of rivalry.

But all this was creating new problems. What was to be Darren's legal relationship to the family? Should they adopt him into the Kaley family?

Somehow that did not seem right. A change of name—for a little black boy to become a member of a Jewish family. No. Name and religion must not be confused in this matter of love, for such changes would only complicate the life of this small boy when he grew up. A celebrity like Sammy Davis, Jr., might opt to become a Jew; it was far too great a responsibility to throw upon the Kaleys to force such a decision.

But the time was approaching when the decision must be faced, because certain legal problems had to be worked out, at the behest of the authorities and the welfare agency. Darren's status had to be clarified so that moneys could keep coming in for his support.

By the end of 1973 the matter became pressing, if only in a legal manner. The Kaleys were happy; Stefanie was doing well in her graduate program. Lou Kaley had been promoted. Mrs. Kaley had found a most congenial part-time position to keep her hand in as bookkeeper. The Dorskys were pleased with the little boy, and he was now able to help with some chores, as he learned the family's habits and needs. Alisa was making remarkable improvement at our school, and some of us at least suspected that part of the reason for it was the "little brother" who had come into her life to give her something more to think about than her own problems.

In the spring of 1974 a decision was forthcoming about Darren's legal position, and all of us at the school and the Kaley household, except Darren, were a little nervous about it. For under New York law, at the end of two years in foster care, a child's case is reviewed by a judge. The judge then decides the child's fate. The two-year period had long passed for Darren, and the court called a hearing. This was the latest in a series of hearings at which various judges had put aside the matter of Darren Dillard over the years, because of various unsettling circumstances, such as the fire.

But now there was to be some more permanent action. Some of the social workers were not at all sure it was healthy for a small black boy to be growing up with a white Jewish family, and they raised the question. We learned of that indirectly. There was nothing in the world we could do about it—the social workers had their own ways and their own access to case histories. The fact that social workers never came to the park to see Darren in action on the baseball diamond, or to watch him wrestling with his friends in the den, or to see the love in Mrs. Kaley's eyes as she cut him a piece of cake—these were not matters that could be translated into legal terms.

The custody of Darren *was* a legal matter.

For six years, Darren's mother had lived in the backdrops of his life. Although she was known to have voiced her hope that he was happy, she never acted on her feelings and came to see him. But that did not dispose of the legal problems involved in relationships between a ward of the court and a natural mother. The mother still had the right to take back her child, if she could prove herself capable of exercising that right.

So in March, 1974, one day the Kaleys received a letter telling them that it was advisable for them to appear in court to discuss the life of the small black boy who had become so much a part of their family. Alarmed, Stefanie called Darren's own social worker and was advised of the procedures, and was told that Darren's mother had also been advised to present whatever material she wished to offer on the situation.

On the day in question the Kaleys and Stefanie went to court in New York City. They entered the big marble building, took the elevator to the courtroom floor, entered the proper room, sat down as directed, and waited.

In her best dress, Stefanie sat on the edge of the hard bench and watched all the people coming into the courtroom. The door was open, and she could see passersby outside. Each time a black woman appeared, she started; could this one be Darren's mother? She looked straight ahead each time.

"I don't want to meet her," she said. "I don't want anything to do with her."

They sat, and they waited. Half an hour went by, and then a familiar face appeared. It was Mr. Forman, our social worker from the Universal Association, and he had come to represent the agency in the court hearing. Stefanie asked if Darren's mother had checked in.

"Don't worry about that, Stefanie," said the man. "I would be very surprised if she appeared at all." He looked into the folder under his hand. "No. She has taken no interest and its been—let's see now—six years. Almost certainly she has decided not to make any contest or to show any interest at all. I can almost guarantee that she will not show up."

The doubt still lingered, but it was much diminished, and Stefanie felt well enough to look around her, more in interest than in fear.

Mr. Forman paused, looked around swiftly, and smiled. "I'll tell you something I probably shouldn't," he said. "We made a lot of tries to get hold of the lady. Then, you know what? She had her telephone number changed. We haven't been able to get in touch with her at all. And she didn't respond to our registered letter."

Suddenly Stefanie felt much, much better.

But only for a moment.

For Mr. Forman was talking again, to her father.

"I hope you can make a good case, Mr. Kaley, if you wish to keep that child. I am afraid the judge is going to wonder about a black Protestant child in a white Jewish family."

"I don't see the problem, sir."

Mr. Forman shook his head and mumbled. Almost immediately he raised a new issue.

"What about adoption? The judge might feel better if you talked about adoption."

"I don't feel that we should adopt the child," Mr. Kaley said. "It simply would be too awkward for him. Too much to explain at this point in his life."

"Perhaps you are right. But I know the judge likes adoptions. I hope you'll be able to keep him on your terms . . ." He sounded very doubtful.

Well, thought Stefanie, why not adopt Darren? She would adopt him if they would let her. She was twenty-one that year. Why not? But she knew, when she considered it, that she had no visible means of caring for the boy. She was dependent on her family still, and any decision that involved such tremendous responsiblity and expense must be made by her mother and father. She also had her own professional and social plans to consider.

So the court proceeding began. The judge entered the room and all stood for him, while the bailiff murmured the prescribed formula for entrance. And court opened.

The judge had the case before him. He had read the report from the agency. He did not know much about Human Resources School, but he asked a few swift, intelligent questions, and nodded his head, satisfied that Darren was getting as fine an education as he could have.

Then the judge addressed himself to the question of the boy himself. The case worker knew, and had written, that the Kaleys were fine foster parents. Darren lived in an atmosphere of love, as well as in a room that met the minimum requirements for sleeping space, and then some.

"Now what about adoption?" the judge asked. Mr. Forman had been right, after all.

"Sir," said Mr. Kaley, "we do not feel at this time that we want to adopt the boy. We have all grown to love him, but there are certain personal factors. First of all, I am forty-five years old and my wife almost the same age. If something were to happen to me it is conceivable that the boy could become a burden . . ."

The judge nodded. "Go on."

"As it is, Darren is assured of care and education at the expense of the welfare authorities. I am not sure that I could offer such great assurances from my own pocket."

The judge nodded again.

"There is another matter," said Mr. Kaley. "Darren has a fine chance in life. The doctors say that in time they can correct his appearance so that he will look almost completely normal. But it is very expensive. He must have a number of plastic surgery operations, over a period of years. Even at today's prices they will surely cost more than any average family could afford. We cannot afford so much, and yet the boy is entitled to that chance in life."

"I agree with you," the judge said. Then he turned to the social worker.

"I want you to get in touch with this woman, his mother," he said. "She has shown no interest in this boy or his welfare for six years. I think that is time enough. Now she must sign the papers to give up all future claims. We are not going to have this good family harried, or in any way disturbed in their work of human charity."

"Mr. Kaley," he said, "I want you to know that this court appreciates what you have done and what you propose to do. It is only proper that you be supported in this by the state. I am not concerned with adoption or with any other purely legal procedures. I am concerned with this boy's welfare, and from what I see here and have learned, I am very pleased to ask you if you would wish to continue custody of him indefinitely under the present status."

"We would, sir," said Lou Kaley.

"Then so be it," said the judge, and he banged down his gavel.

21

Happiness

The Kaleys left the court as happy as a family could be, and hurried home to tell the Dorskys and Darren what had occurred. In the days just prior to the hearing they had tried to keep Darren from learning what was going on, but a word here and one there —and that eager mind taking it all in. He had known. The night before the hearing he had spoken up to Stefanie.

"Tomorrow you go to court, don't you? About me?"

She had admitted that it was so. Now she could

rush into the house, and find Darren just home from school, throw her arms around his neck, and cry a little because she was so pleased at the outcome of the hearing.

So the year 1974 was an important one for Darren; it established his place in the Kaley household, and although nothing was ever said, that court appearance had settled matters once and for all. Stefanie no longer had her nightmares or her fears that Darren would be lost to her. The judge had decreed that the foster-family relationship was to continue, and there was no reason it should be ended until Darren was ready to strike out for himself in the world. That meant he would go through high school, and through college.

For of course, this was what we were all beginning to realize about Darren. It had come slowly—for when he came to us, a shy little mouse, he seemed to be as badly handicapped as any spinal case or wheelchair child we had. Now, after two operations, and his growth and development in the Kaley household, the doctors were telling us that they could make him so nearly normal that he could soon go out into the general stream of American life.

This *was* a challenge. It was the best news any of us connected with the Human Resources School could imagine. For it came right down to our reason for being—the establishment of the best possible conditions of life for those wonderful children who started out with handicaps. And here, right with us, was the little boy who with enough care and attention could be moved right back into mainstream.

But—it was going to take some doing.

We consulted, the Kaleys and I, with various doctors at North Shore Community Hospital in Manhasset, and we came up with a medical and surgical program for Darren. He was going to have to have a number of operations. Most taxing and long lasting would be the procedures to build the non-existent cheekbone on the left side of his face. Every two years until he was eighteen years old he would have to go into the hospital for an operation to change the artificial cheek bone to meet the growth of his head and the other side of his face.

During August of 1974 he had two more surgical operations, one on his eye socket, to strengthen the muscle and tissue so that it would hold the eye in firmly and one on his ear. The eye operation was needed, for, by school's end, the eye was still coming out occasionally—as on the basketball floor—but this operation was scheduled to finish that job.

And then the arduous process of building that ear would be continued again in 1975. However, even by the end of December it was really beginning to look like an ear, although still a foreshortened and not very pretty one. Every two or three months Darren would have to go to the hospital for another bit of surgery.

To a boy any less bright or optimistic, it might have been too much of a blow, this constant battle with surgery. But Darren knew somehow that it was part of his salvation, and he bore the pain and the trouble of it without a whimper. As for school, he sailed through kindergarten, managing the class as much as the teacher would let him, and in the fall of 1974 he entered Eileen Singleton's first grade.

But already, that autumn, we were talking to the

superintendent of Syosset's schools about Darren. Stefanie took him down to the administration building one day, and they made arrangements for him to visit the school near the house, where the Swaris boys and his other pals attended. They went over there one afternoon—and were promptly mobbed in the hall by all Darren's friends, who somehow seemed to sense that he was coming.

"Whatcha doin' here, Darren?" asked Scott.

"Yeah," chimed in Joe, the big kid who had rubbed sand in Darren's hair that day in the park.

Darren looked up at Stefanie.

"Maybe I'll come here to school next year," he said.

"That would be great," said Scott. "Why not this year?"

"Don't be in too big a hurry, boys," said Stefanie. "Darren's got some catching up to do."

But when they left that afternoon, and Stefanie asked Darren if he really wanted to go to the neighborhood school, he gave it all away.

"Want to?" he asked. "I'm going to. Our school is great but I really can't *play* with anybody."

And of course that was just the reason that it was nearly time for Darren to be off in the main stream of life. We were going to do everything we could to make that transition possible. This is the destiny for all our children.

While Darren was visiting class at the Syosset school, the teacher and the principal watched more carefully than one might have thought. Later they told Dick and Eileen Singleton that they were really surprised at the way Darren managed to fit himself into the class when he was there only for that afternoon as a visitor. Obviously they had feared that his color or his handicap, or both, might go against him. None of the children of the first grade payed the slightest attention. Nor did they give more than cursory attention to the eye and the ear. Part of the reason must have been that so many of these children had played with Darren, or had at least seen him around the neighborhood. He was just another kid to them—the way it ought to be.

There were many consultations in many quarters that fall. Stefanie kept in contact with Eileen Singleton about the things she found out about the work being done in the Syosset schools. In this way Eileen could be sure that her particular teaching program for Darren could be adjusted, if necessary, so that he would fit in the next year.

Very little change was necessary. Our school at Human Resources is at par, at least, with all the public schools around Long Island. Darren had a bright and inquiring mind, and he was not going to have any trouble adjusting. Eileen could see that in the beginning of the year.

22

Preparation

It was our self-appointed job in 1974 and 1975 to make Darren ready to go out into the wide world that he would face when he joined the other youngsters of second grade in public school in the fall of 1975.

Quite naturally we had already done one thing for Darren simply by having him in our school: we had tapped the springs of human compassion in this small boy. And nowhere was that fact more apparent than in Eileen Singleton's first grade class.

We had nine students in first grade in the fall of 1974, and by this time Darren was the least disabled of the lot. For example we had Nadia, with brittle bones, and Rita, who has spina bifida; Pansy, a spina bifida, Michel, an arthrogyrasis, and Claudine, who is also in a walker and a wheel chair, and Peggy with her neck in a brace.

Darren came in the first day, announced that he was going to be Eileen's assistant, and began doing just that. He organized the other children, assisted them with coats and hats—helped them so vigorously that Eileen worried lest he break a bone or hurt another without meaning to.

Then he helped set up the routine, which is so essential for an orderly day in our school. For when the children arrive in the morning on their buses, they are all excited and ready to go. But it is not quite so easy. They must be helped to get out of their things —but not helped too much, for it is our policy to encourage self-help.

And then their medications and their "changing" must be managed. Those children whose illnesses make them incontinent must be taken to the nurse's office for diaper and prosthetic changes when necessary; the teacher must know precisely what she is doing. And in first grade it was not very long before Mr. Assistant Teacher was ready to remind Eileen if she forgot anything at all.

Immediately, Darren was the star of the class. The girls quarreled over him. When it came time for rest, whose mat would be next to his? Sometimes it was one, sometimes it was another. He was a fickle one, and one day he was promising to marry one girl and then it would be another.

I have not mentioned it much in this book, because it is so completely unimportant in our particular world, but the question of race and color never entered into anyone's thinking at the school. One day Darren would be proposing marriage to a white girl and the next to a black, and the little girls felt precisely the same way that he did, that we all did: who cared about such nonessentials? It is only in the outside world that there is caring about these things.

Not that we did not prepare Darren for this, too. Stefanie was best of all, for she used to think it was necessary to have some formal discussions about racial issues. (She was quite right.) But with her attitude and his, the talks usually ended up in laughter, with both of them rolling on the floor. Here is one such talk that Stefanie described:

Stefanie: You know Darren, you are black and I am white.

Darren: I am? Then why am I so light and why are you so dark? (This was just after a summer in which Stefanie had been playing tennis nearly every day.)

Stefanie: Now listen, I am trying to tell you something important.

Darren: Then why are Scott and Chris darker than I am? Are they black?

Stefanie: No, they are Ceylonese. Like Indian people."

Darren: Are Indians dark?

Stefanie: Yes. Some of them are very dark.

Darren: Darker than the Swarises?

Stefanie: Much darker.

Darren: Then why aren't they black?

Stefanie: Oh, you're impossible! (tickle)

Darren: (Laughter.) Stop that!

They collapse on the floor of the den and wrestle.

But sometimes she was more serious and managed to explain to Darren that in life he was going to meet people who would be mean to him because of his color. She also made it a point to take out books from the library showing blacks and whites together. He learned.

And it would ever be so, for in a family like the Kaleys where love reigned supreme, no real thought of color or shape could possibly exist. Luckily for all of us it was almost as fine in terms of love at school.

Each day in Eileen's class there would be some new triumph for Darren, whether it be academic or social. He was unquestionably the star of the class, and it was about all Dick Switzer could do from keeping him from becoming the star of the school. We had to be careful, there were egos involved—not just the egos of other students, but we could not afford to let Darren get a swelled head, in his own behalf. So he had to be stepped on. And luckily as small boys will do, he managed to get himself into trouble from time to time through his exuberance.

One day, when Eileen had specifically told Darren to be very careful in wheeling the other children of the class about in their chairs, he began pushing Nadia so fast that she nearly cried. Suddenly Darren cried out.

"Ouch," he said. "I wrecked my hand."

"And a good thing, too," said Eileen sternly, "before you turned Nadia out of her chair and let her hurt herself."

"But I hurt my finger," pleaded Darren, aghast at

the unsympathetic world he found around him.

"Your own fault, Darren. Be more careful."

But of course Eileen could not stay angry. And he might indeed have hurt himself. So she sent him up to see Judy, who looked over the offending finger, gave it an exploratory feel, and put an ice bag on it. He wore the ice bag all afternoon long, making sure it was replenished several times.

Then Darren went home. Next morning he reappeared at school triumphantly, wearing a splint on his finger.

"See," he said, holding up the finger. "I broke it. And my father took me to the doctor and he put a splint on it. See. I told you so."

But it was a lesson nonetheless. And in the future he kept his fingers out of the wheels of the wheelchairs.

He was all boy, too, and while he loved the girls, one at a time and all together, in his mind girls had their place, and it was very definite. Darren had a coat that was the same color and same general cut as little Claudine's coat, although there was about four sizes difference between them, and his was a boy's coat and hers a girl's (which meant they buttoned on different sides). One day in the rush of going home, someone grabbed Darren's coat and flung it on little Claudine before she got into her wheelchair and headed for the bus. There was Darren, left behind, cleaning up for Eileen that day.

Suddenly he realized how late it was and grabbed his coat. But it was Claudine's coat, he saw with disgust. And Darren flung it back on its hook and shouted that he was not going to wear any girl's coat home in the bus and disgrace himself.

Crisis. It was a cold February day, and Darren must have a coat. Claudine's was the only coat left, and he must take it. That was authority—which Eileen summoned with some effort.

No.

All right, then, he must wear the coat out to the heated bus and get in the bus, and then he could put the coat down and when he got home he could take it in and explain to his mother.

Fine.

Crisis resolved. And Darren went home.

But Claudine, who was a little scatterbrained at times, kept losing things and taking things. One day she took Darren's sweater home—either by mistake or suffering from pangs of love. He was furious, and next day he took Claudine's doll home and refused to return it until she promised she would leave his coat and his sweater alone. She promised.

By springtime, we were ready for another round of hospitalization. One day in May, Stefanie came home in the afternoon and packed up Darren's little suitcase. He knew what that meant.

"Not again," he said mournfully.

"Come on. Let's go get a hamburger," she said.

That was the signal. A hamburger always meant —well not always, but a hamburger and the suitcase —a trip to the hospital. This time it was the ear again.

"Unhhhhh," he said. "I'm not sure I want to eat."

But that was the end of his plaint. They went to a hamburger place and had big sandwiches and milkshakes, and then it was over to North Shore Hospital.

"You know, Steffie," he said, as they pulled into

the parking lot, "I *hate* it when they put the mask on you."

But in he went, for a blood test and a final checkup that night, and surgery in the morning.

The next day, after her classes, Stefanie met her mother at the hospital. There he was, at noon, still quiet in the recovery room. He came to while she was holding his hand.

"Hey, Steffie," he grinned. "They didn't use the mask this time. And guess what? We learned the neatest game." He was referring to the pediatric ward, where he had spent the night. "You take these old hypodermics and use them for squirt guns . . . Boy. . . ."

She shuddered, and then had to struggle with her conscience. Should she tell the nurse? In a week's time Darren, bandages and all, was back at school.

By this time at our school, Dr. Marie Meier, our School Psychologist, had observed Darren in a dozen situations at school, and she told Dick Switzer that we could all be proud, for she would take bets that Darren was going to do just fine in the outside world. He had come to the school an insecure child, and one we worried about a good deal. He was now getting ready to leave, advanced for his age, able to hold his own in any situation that he could be expected to resolve, not aggressive but able to stand up for himself. And—Dr. Meier brought this to our minds—little Darren had to be given all kinds of credit for the strength he was showing in the face of the medical and surgical program before him.

23
The Birthday Party

In spite of setting up the chain of events that would lead to Darren's entrance into the outside world by going into Syosset public schools, the Kaleys and I worried a good deal about our decision early in 1975.

"You know, Hank," said Dick Switzer one day, "we talk an awful lot about mainstreaming because it sounds so very good. Here we are taking cripples—the outcasts of society—and bringing them right into the center of American life. That's what we say. But are we?"

"What do you mean?"

"I mean are these people really going to be able to hack it in the other world? The competition is pretty rough."

We had several reasons to think in those terms. One was the worsening of the economy in 1974 and 1975; when that happens the handicapped are last in and first out on the payroll.

Over the years we had also had some experiences in Human Resources with people who had been trained in other schools, and after months and years of quiet desperation had found solace by working for us. For we *understand* the problems of the handicapped and our organization is equipped to deal with them in a competent, sympathetic, but no-nonsense manner. A few failures, in the matter of sending young people out into the world of the physically fit, might set back the cause of rehabilition, not to mention the possibility of harm to a youngster who did not make it on the outside.

So, would Darren make it? That was the question we had to answer for ourselves even as we put the wheels in motion that would take him away from us.

Why not? He was getting all the care that he could possibly have under any situation. The Kaleys and the doctors and nurses had established a sensible physical rehabilitation program for him, and he was taking it so well we could hardly believe it. When Darren was eighteen years old, he would be ready for college, just at the time that subsistence payments ran out. By that time he would have a fully developed left ear, his eye would be firmly anchored in a socket that should be indistinguishable from the other, his cheekbone would be built up so there would be no sagging in his face. In other words, he would be, on the outside, a complete human being.

Luckily, on the inside he was even better off. He was intelligent, willing, and he had a poise that was remarkable considering his background. He was a natural leader. In fact, when Stefanie suggested to an upper echelon administrator of the local school district that she worried about the problem of his changing schools, he just laughed at her. He lives on the Kaleys' block and had seen Darren several times in situations there. He knew Darren by that time.

"Don't you worry about Darren," the man said. "One of these days he's going to be the mayor of Syosset."

So as the months of 1975 slipped by, we worried less and less about Darren's ability to make the change, for when the administrator in Syosset labeled him a potential politician he was quite right—Dick Switzer also called Darren "the mayor of Human Resources."

He went sailing on through first grade, getting his reading and subtraction and his addition down as well as anyone. He was going to have no trouble at all with the academic change to public school, Eileen Singleton assured us.

And as for the social transition, why Darren had already made it with no more damage or ruffling than that headful of sand he got one afternoon. By midwinter he already knew many of the children in the first grade at Syosset—the ones he would join the next year —and the boys at least accepted him without a tremor. No more strange looks at the eye or the ear. No complaints. There were a few black children in the school, and a variety of religions represented—some Protestants, some Catholics, and a number of Jewish boys and girls, for this section of Syosset is mixed. The level of tolerance was very high.

Thinking of that, of course, we had to think further to the junior high and high school level. But we could not play God. By the time Darren reached junior high, his face repairs would be very nearly finished. He would simply have to take his chances. Given his character and the remarkable development in two years, we had no worries. Darren's birthday party in February was a climax, in a way, to all we had been thinking and saying.

Actually, there were two birthday parties. One was held at home with the Swaris boys and a half dozen of Darren's other playmates from around the neighborhood, and Mary Switzer, Dick's daughter, who is his "best girl." There was spaghetti and meatballs and ice cream cake, and candy to eat. Darren got a new jacket and some other clothes, a toy gas station that Lou Kaley had to assemble, a football, a book and two record albums. They played pin-the-tail-on-the-donkey and tag.

When the lunch had been served and they had their ice cream and cake, Darren blew out all his eight candles (one to grow on) in one big breath. Darren wore a crown, and all the other children had paper hats. By the time the cake came they were a smeary group, for Stefanie and her mother had made up favors of candy for everyone—M&Ms, peanutclusters, and Chuckles. And everyone either sang a song or recited a poem.

School had its own party. The children insisted on that. Eileen Singleton was absent that day, so I supervised. It was a more restrained affair, as school parties must be, but a fine success. We had vanilla and chocolate cupcakes with icing, and Darren had a candle on his cupcake. We listened to records and everybody had to dance, including me. Suddenly somebody remembered that we had no party hats. . . .

"You can't have a party without hats," said Darren.

So we began scouring around for hats, and sure enough, in the nursery school we found the collection of hats that parents send in from time to time. They are always on hand for our children. There was an old top hat, a fedora, and a derby, and a fine collection of ladies' hats. So we all put on funny hats and laughed at one another while we ate our cake and the substitute teacher told stories.

That was Darren's birthday, and the separation of the two parties is in a way very indicative of the life he has lived until now. It has been a busy life, and in its own way a very successful one. An unwanted crippled child came to us in 1972 out of institutions and foster homes where love was at a premium. Here at the residence, he found acceptance and a new life—one so definitely endangered by the fire that burned the house and caused us to abandon our whole plan of school residency.

In a way you could say that the fire was a cleansing agent, and that out of its ashes arose a Phoenix child. For had it not been for the fire, Darren would never have gone to stay with the Kaleys, he would never have known the complete love that only a family can bring, and he would have been at best not more than half of what he is.

And I have watched our Phoenix grow and prosper in this atmosphere of love, showing through his own return of love how a little child can strengthen the bonds within a family. I have seen Alisa Kaley prosper because of Darren's coming, and Stefanie has told me how it has made her more responsible and helped her prepare for the career she has chosen. The Phoenix has done well.

The story of the Phoenix child, the story of Darren and the Kaleys, is in its way a modern miracle, and yet how old. For no matter our growth in sophistication and the trappings of an atomic society, the age-old truths remain. And the greatest of these is love. Little black disfigured Darren Dillard has taught me that.

His was a love that was always building up, so like our love for our disabled children. It puts some kind of beauty into every life it touches. It makes life seem more worthwhile to everyone into whose eye it looks. Its words are benedictions. Its every breath is full of inspiration.